CREATIVE WAYS TO HELP CHILDREN REGULATE AND MANAGE ANGER

by the same author

Creative Ways to Help Children Manage Anxiety
Ideas and Activities for Working Therapeutically with Worried Children and Their Families
Dr. Fiona Zandt and Dr. Suzanne Barrett
Illustrated by Richy K. Chandler
Foreword by Dr. Karen Cassiday
ISBN 978 1 78775 094 4
eISBN 978 1 78775 095 1

Creative Ways to Help Children Manage Big Feelings
A Therapist's Guide to Working with Preschool and Primary Children
Dr. Fiona Zandt and Dr. Suzanne Barrett
Foreword by Associate Professor Lesley Bretherton
ISBN 978 1 78592 074 5
eISBN 978 1 78450 487 8

of related interest

How to Be Angry
Strategies to Help Kids Express Anger Constructively
Signe Whitson
Illustrated by Adam A. Freeman
Foreword by Dr. Lori Desautels
ISBN 978 1 83997 130 3
eISBN 978 1 83997 131 0

Starving the Anger Gremlin
A Cognitive Behavioural Therapy Workbook on Anger Management for Young People
Kate Collins-Donnelly
ISBN 978 1 84905 286 3
eISBN 978 0 85700 621 9

Starving the Anger Gremlin for Children Aged 5–9
A Cognitive Behavioural Therapy Workbook on Anger Management
Kate Collins-Donnelly
ISBN 978 1 84905 493 5
eISBN 978 0 85700 885 5

Anger the Ancient Warrior
A Story and Workbook with CBT Activities to Master Your Anger
Sarah Trueman and Sara Godoli
Illustrated by Dorian Cottereau
ISBN 978 1 78775 368 6
eISBN 978 1 78775 369 3

CREATIVE WAYS TO HELP CHILDREN REGULATE AND MANAGE ANGER

IDEAS AND ACTIVITIES FOR WORKING WITH ANGER AND EMOTIONAL REGULATION

DR. FIONA ZANDT

Foreword By Dr. Lorri A. Yasenik

Illustrations By Richy K. Chandler

Jessica Kingsley Publishers

London and Philadelphia

First published in Great Britain in 2024 Jessica Kingsley Publishers
An imprint of John Murray Press

1

A CIP catalogue record for this title is available from the British Library and the Library of Congress

ISBN 978 1 83997 556 1
eISBN 978 1 83997 557 8

Printed and bound in Great Britain by TJ Books Ltd

Jessica Kingsley Publishers' policy is to use papers that are natural, renewable and recyclable products
and made from wood grown in sustainable forests. The logging and manufacturing processes
are expected to conform to the environmental regulations of the country of origin.

Jessica Kingsley Publishers
Carmelite House
50 Victoria Embankment
London EC4Y 0DZ

www.jkp.com

John Murray Press
Part of Hodder & Stoughton Ltd
An Hachette Company

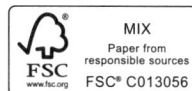

MIX
Paper from
responsible sources
FSC® C013056

Printed and bound in Great Britain by
TJ Books Limited, Padstow, Cornwall

To Charli, with all my love.

And to James, Joe, Chris and Edie,
for continually challenging me to walk new paths.

Contents

Foreword by Lorri A. Yasenik **11**

Acknowledgements **13**

Preface **15**

1. **Before You Start** **17**
   Why anger arises   17
   Anger and the development of regulation   19
   The neuroscience of regulation   21
   Regulation and the therapeutic relationship   23
   Anger and diagnosis   23
   Theoretical frameworks and evidence base   25
   On language   26
   Knowing your own feelings about anger   27
   Regulation for therapists   29
   The role of play and using playful activities   30
   The importance of grownups   32
   Finding new paths   35

2. **First Sessions** **39**
   Finding the balance   39
   First sessions with children   41
     Setting up the space for children   41
     Assessing a child's emotional awareness and regulation skills   43
     Assessing coping and calming   44
   First sessions with grownups   45
     Exploring grownups' own experiences of anger   45
     Understanding grownups' responses and reflective capacity   47
     General family functioning   50
     Openness to different ideas   51
   Keeping first sessions play-based   52

ACTIVITIES FOR THE FIRST SESSIONS

My anger is…   54

What's bugging you?   55

The shape of my anger   56

Rainbow pom-pom feelings   58

Angry puppet stories   60

Bang it out   61

Inside and outside elastics jump   62

Inside and outside noticing dice   64

3. Moving into Therapy   67

Making sense of it all and coming up with a plan   67

Working in a way that fits for the child and family   68

   Understanding what the child needs   68

   Understanding what the grownups need   72

Goal-setting and treatment planning   77

Tracking progress through ongoing assessment   78

4. Calming the Body   81

Developing calming and self-soothing routines   82

Calming in sessions   83

Calming and coping strategies for day-to-day life   84

Increasing calming strategies   86

ACTIVITIES FOR CALMING THE BODY

Pit stops   88

Calming animal shapes   90

Taking your emotional temperature   92

Breathing sensory bag   94

I'm on your team   96

CALM for you, CALM for me   98

My magic bag   100

Umbrellas for angry moments   102

5. Understanding and Expressing Anger 105

What we want children to understand about anger   106

Handout: Understanding anger   108

Recognizing anger   109

   Recognizing how stretched the child is and seeing the build-up   110

   Noticing body signs   112

   Understanding the feelings underneath anger   113

   Remembering that anger will pass   114

   Recognizing patterns   115

When anger doesn't come into the room   115

ACTIVITIES THAT HELP CHILDREN NOTICE AND NAME ANGER

My anger song   117

Splat anger   118

Getting in the tank   119

Tunnelling through the feeling   121

Angry balloon feelings   122

Kindness binoculars   124

Sitting with all my feelings   126

How stretched are you today?   128

Magnifying feelings   130

Unsafe animals   131

Understanding anger dice game   132

Different feeling parts   134

Baby babushka feelings   136

Seeing the other feelings in my anger   139

Clouds of anger   141

The washing machine   142

Spinning anger   144

See it differently   146

Who's that knocking?   147

Getting comfortable with uncomfortable feelings and thoughts   149

6. **Responding to Anger in the Room and Supporting Grownups to Respond** **151**

Responding to anger in sessions   151

Setting limits in therapy and helping grownups to do so   153

Helping grownups to regulate their children using HOLDS   154

H is for Having a moment to connect with your own feelings and look after yourself   155

O is for Organizing the child's feelings, as well as the situation   156

L is for Looking for the feelings underneath   157

D is for Doing the things that are regulating   158

S is for Speaking after the child and grownup are regulated   158

Considerations when using this model   161

When grownups don't get it right   162

When therapists need to use HOLDS   163

ACTIVITIES TO SUPPORT FAMILIES WITH REGULATION

Handout: HOLDS for your child   165

Talk, don't talk   166

Rupture and repair with Play-Doh   168

7. **Thinking About Anger** **169**

How and when to use cognitive strategies   169

Helpful concepts around thoughts   172

Problem-solving   174

P is for Pausing and taking a breath   175

I is for thinking of an Idea to try and giving it a go   175

K is for Keep going for long enough to see if it works   176

S is for Stop and try something else if need be   176

ACTIVITIES FOR HELPING CHILDREN THINK ABOUT ANGER

Handout: Problem-solving for kids   178

Lucky dip choices   179

Different roads   180

Problem-solving puppets   182

Anger word match   183

Sticky thoughts with sticky tape   185

Thinking and feeling brain hats   187

In and out of my hands with anger   189

8. Choosing and Doing What Is Important. 191

Choosing and doing what is important for children   191

And for grownups   193

ACTIVITIES THAT HELP CHILDREN AND GROWNUPS
CHOOSE AND DO WHAT IS IMPORTANT

Heading toward what is important   195

Holding on to what is important   197

Route recalculation   199

Toward ladders and away from snakes   200

9. When Things Get Tricky 203

Developing a plan   204

Legal and ethical responsibilities   206

A word about working online   207

10. Dealing with Common Triggers. 209

ACTIVITIES THAT ADDRESS COMMON TRIGGERS FOR ANGER

Changing plans with Connect 4   212

Slimy messy mistakes   213

Holding on to the shoulds   214

Final Thoughts 217

References 219

Foreword

Anger is one of our strongest emotions. It is essential but at the same time few people feel comfortable in the midst of an angry person. Anger is hard for parents to accept in their children and difficult for many practitioners to address in therapy. It's often an unwelcome expression that evokes the desire to "shut it down." But what is useful about the complex emotion *anger*? This essential text on getting to know anger, begins with *you* and your own feelings about anger and then identifies the many roles anger plays in our lives.

The neuroscience of regulation is also addressed in a way that both practitioners and caregivers will find useful. Polyvagal theory (Porges 2017) and window of tolerance and emotion regulation (Siegel 2020) are helpful theories to underpin various interventions to assist children and youth to understand, manage and express strong feelings. Identifying a child's anger and providing language and understanding of a child's relationship with strong feelings is the first step to working more deeply with the child's emotions and autonomic nervous system. The neuroception of safety in the counselling space is critical when working with threat responses such as anger and aggression, as this allows for the greater awareness of proprioception (the awareness of where our bodies are in space) and interoception (the awareness of what is going on in our bodies).

This book is a useful resource for a wide range of child therapists and is well suited to play therapy. Play therapists work with children and youth using a variety of play materials and are usually trained to utilize a number of theoretical orientations. Those working with children are familiar with beginning where the *child is at* and allowing the child to show and tell about their feelings, thoughts and experiences. This book emphasizes tailoring activities to the *child's* needs and personal ways of experiencing anger. The described activities require the therapist to consider their use of self on the directiveness continuum as directive prompts and specific materials are suggested. Regarding the Play Therapy Dimensions Model (Yasenik and Gardner 2012), the interventions move from Quadrant II (Open Discussion and Exploration, where the therapist provides a direct invitation or addresses a topic directly) to Quadrant III (Non-intrusive Responding or child-led play) to Quadrant IV (Co-facilitation, where the therapist is actively joining and adding to the play). The activities invite a lead-follow-lead approach. Play-based practitioners will be well equipped to make use of the ideas outlined as they will benefit from having a range of materials available, including art making, puppets, miniatures, Play-Doh, sandtray and games. Alternative materials are suggested throughout, making the activities accessible regardless of the context in which you work. The activities in the book can also be modified to suit a particular child and preferably include caregivers.

It is important to include caregivers as they also need ways to regulate in order to be available to co-regulate their child. Increasing parent/child attunement assists parents to accurately read and then sensitively respond to their child's cues. A lovely metaphor of a well-worn, well-traveled path is initially used to introduce parents to our automatic neural pathways. It is the beginning of considering what it would mean to take another, less known and possibly less comfortable path to create new pathways and positive change. Caregivers are also encouraged to explore their own experiences of anger. The family focus removes the child from the identified problem and shifts working with anger to a more universal human experience.

Each chapter has some wonderfully useful and engaging activities, and although the point is made that many activities are directive in nature, the text is also sensitive to the top-down/bottom-up brain science concepts of how to work with specific children. It requires the therapist to understand the young person in front of them and to purposefully conceptualize how to engage with that child. The activities take into account mind/body responses and go beyond a traditional cognitive behavioral focus. Two helpful acronyms, one for connecting and checking in (referred to as HOLDS) and one for problem-solving (PIKS) are described and broken down for the practitioner to use with both children and caregivers.

Overall, *Creative Ways to Help Children Regulate and Manage Anger* is a great addition to the literature for child therapists working with anger and emotion regulation. It highlights the practitioner, caregiver and child. It is practical and thoughtfully uses question prompts and case vignettes to bring the topic alive. It leads the practitioner to explore the underbelly of anger.

Lorri A. Yasenik, PhD, CPT-S, RPT-S
Director of the Rocky Mountain Play Therapy Institute in Calgary, Canada

Acknowledgements

I am incredibly grateful for the support of my colleagues Suzanne Barrett, Nicole Francke, Sarah Francke, Sue Ellis and Emma Menkinoska for their thoughtful comments on this manuscript.

I am also incredibly thankful for the ongoing support of Jane Evans, Laura Savage, and the team at Jessica Kingsley Publishers. I am humbled and grateful to be supporting the learning of other therapists and, in turn, to be helping more children and families.

Thank you to my beautiful friends and family for all your support, both more generally and in the writing of this book. Thanks especially to Faith, Megan and Renai for always believing in me and to James, Joseph, Christian and Edith, for their ongoing love and support.

Most of all, I am grateful to the inspiring children and families who have allowed me to be a small part of their journey. Thank you for challenging me to find playful ways and helping me co-create these activities as we walk new paths together.

Preface

This book is intended for mental health professionals and is not a substitute for clinical training or ongoing supervision. This grounding is essential in helping you to apply the suggestions in this book to your practice, knowing which are likely to be helpful for the children and families you see.

Throughout this book I have attempted to acknowledge other authors whenever I am conscious of their influence. I have also shared relevant books and research where appropriate, noting what is useful clinically rather than endeavoring to summarize all of the available literature. Study in this area is ever increasing, and the ongoing developments in the field mean that neither the author nor the publisher can ensure that the material contained within is up to date at the time of reading.

CHAPTER 1

BEFORE YOU START

Anger is a complicated emotion: perhaps more than any other it evokes incredibly strong feelings, thoughts and beliefs in others. And yet, anger is an emotion like all others. It is normal and valuable. Everyone experiences it at times, and, like all feelings, it passes. While this may seem obvious, it seems to be something that we forget when it comes to children. There is something about seeing their child angry that tends to make grownups very uncomfortable, anxiously avoiding this or responding in kind and quickly shutting it down. Anger can also mask other feelings, such as anxiety or sadness.

This book is for therapists who work with children who have difficulties with anger. It is full of playful ways to help children and their grownups understand anger and manage it differently. This chapter provides some background information about anger and orientates you to the work by encouraging you to reflect on your own relationship with anger and prepare for working with children and their grownups. The following chapters move through first sessions, calming strategies, understanding anger, cognitive approaches and working on common triggers. These chapters contain lots of practical ideas for working with children and families as well as playful therapeutic activities you can use in sessions. Throughout the book you will see a focus on working with families and Chapter 6 focuses on supporting grownups to regulate their child.

It is my hope in writing this book that more child therapists will honor the anger that children bring, carefully sifting through it to find what it is a child is communicating and helping the child's grownups to be with them through this.

Why anger arises

Anger has numerous roles and arises in many different contexts. In this section we explore some of the contexts in which anger arises, examining what this might communicate rather than focusing on the behaviors through which anger is expressed. Looking more deeply helps us to better understand the support a child and family are likely to need.

One of anger's roles is as a protector. It is a strong emotion that helps us to set limits. A child who does not learn to express their anger in an appropriate way is vulnerable, for it is anger that supports us to set boundaries and limits with others. The child who becomes angry in response to being bullied by a peer is, for example, likely to avoid future interactions with that child and may attempt to develop new friendships. Some children have had experiences in which anger has kept them safe in traumatic situations. For those who have experienced moments of powerlessness and vulnerability in their lives, anger may provide a temporary sense of power and control. Indeed, recent meta-analyses have found childhood maltreatment to be associated with increased emotional dysregulation in childhood and adolescence (Gruhn and Compas 2020; Lavi *et al.* 2019).

Anger is also an informer. It helps us to tune in to what is important to us and lets us know when something needs to be different. Putting anger into words and identifying the underlying hurts, anxieties or needs, allows for a better understanding of our own experience and can prompt us to take action. Indeed, the role of anger in facilitating action is important to acknowledge too. The intensity of anger encourages us to notice and explore these feelings, often supporting us to make some different choices.

Sometimes anger is a communicator, letting others know that something is wrong. Young children typically communicate through their behavior, and sometimes anger communicates a child's distress or unmet needs. A child may reflect their distress at some of the challenges within their family through anger outbursts. They may also communicate their need for connection with grownups by behaving in ways that grownups inevitably need to attend to. Children might learn that anger or aggression is a way to communicate distress. For example, Li, Ma and Zhang (2023) reviewed the literature to find that children who were raised in a context of parental conflict were more likely to be aggressive in their own relationships with peers, family members and partners. Anger can help us to understand that a child is struggling in a particular area. For example, a child who becomes overwhelmed and angry when interacting with groups of peers might be communicating that a child is struggling with social interaction and needs support. Identifying these needs, or what Dr. Ross Greene (2014) refers to as lagging skills, is essential if we are to effectively support children.

Anger is often a secondary emotion, with another emotion underlying it. For example, a child who feels worried about getting sick may explode angrily at her brother leaving his tissue on the couch. Anxiety is often expressed through controlling behavior and anger. Similarly children can respond to embarrassment, sadness or shame in an angry manner. Recognizing that there is often another emotion underneath is important. Not only does it allow us to address the underlying emotion more effectively, for most families the emotion underneath is often more understandable and they often feel more empowered to empathize and respond once they learn about the feelings underneath their child's anger.

Sometimes anger is not related to the current experience. It may be directed at someone or something else, despite being expressed in the current moment. For example, a child who has faced a number of stresses at school may become angry at their parents in the afternoon as a way of releasing some of their feelings. Facilitating an exploration to allow for a better understanding of this is essential.

When we are curious about anger and explore what it is telling us we can better understand and meet a child's needs. We can support children to express their anger more appropriately, help them communicate the feelings underneath and approach their anger with a curiosity about what it might mean.

Anger and the development of regulation

It is not possible to talk about anger difficulties without talking about regulation. What children who struggle with anger often lack is the ability to regulate their emotions. Further, emotion regulation is a common goal in our work across a broad range of presentations in which anger and aggression are the central concern. Understanding what emotional regulation is (and isn't) therefore is essential. In this section we explore what emotional regulation is, how it develops, and what we understand about it from neuroscience.

Emotional regulation refers to "the general ability of the mind…to alter the various components of emotional processing" (Siegel 2020, p.333). Put another way, it is our ability to respond to our emotions in a way that is consistent with our values and goals. It is the ability to be angry and still make good choices; the ability to respond thoughtfully instead of simply reacting. Importantly, emotional regulation is not about suppressing feelings or becoming calm, rather it is about leaning in to our feelings and consciously trying to understand these whilst being able to still access those thinking parts of our brain so that we can choose how we respond.

Siegel (2020) describes how children first learn about emotions from the grownups around them, typically their parents, beginning in infancy. How grownups respond to their own emotions, engage in emotion management, model regulation and the emotional climate of the family are all likely to influence the way a child experiences, expresses and regulates emotions (Morris *et al.* 2007). The way in which grownups respond to a child's emotions is likely to be particularly formative. Ideally, when babies and young children experience uncomfortable emotions, such as sadness or anger, the attuned grownup will notice and name this feeling for them, picking them up and soothing them. Importantly, when grownups perceive their baby's emotional response they are activated in parallel, which results in mutual attunement and creates a shared emotional experience, in which grownup and infant become more regulated together. When this process, which is often referred to as co-regulation, is repeated time and time again as the child moves through infancy and toddlerhood into the preschool years, they begin to associate the feelings in their body with the named feeling. They also understand that it is safe to express their feelings and know they can be supported with these.

The experience of being regulated helps children learn to regulate themselves. These early experiences often create a cascade effect, with attachment studies supporting the idea that the pattern of communication with their grownups creates adaptations that shape the development of the child's nervous system and their subsequent interactions (Siegel 2020). Havighurst and Kehoe (2017) note that children who have had their emotions recognized and validated, who are encouraged to talk about their emotions and are supported to regulate their emotions, do better socially and academically. Conversely, children who have experienced unsupportive or dismissive responses are more likely to experience both internalizing and externalizing behavior difficulties. In the context of therapy, therefore, exploring grownups' early experiences of regulating their child as well as their current experience helps us to understand the context for a given child.

Secure attachment fosters emotional regulation, with the child's grownups being present and providing soothing in times of distress and joining with them in moments of joy. This process can be disrupted for a broad range of reasons, even when grownups are available to care for their children without disruption. Some children (and grownups) respond more intensely to emotions than others, which is likely to be a product of both their individual makeup and their experiences. Some children (and grownups) are also more sensitive than others, becoming emotional more readily. Parent-rated temperament has been found to predict psychopathology later in childhood. For example, a recent study by Morales and colleagues (2022) found that higher motor activity in infancy was associated with greater psychopathology in mid to late childhood. Different levels of reactivity in children are likely to elicit different parenting responses and, in turn, parenting practices shape the way in which children respond. The interplay between a child's temperament and their environment therefore continues over time. Parental stress, for example, is also likely to be another key factor in this complex dynamic (McQuillan and Bates 2017). Further, Siegel (2020) notes that a child's experiences, both within their family and social circles and within their broader cultural context, shape the way in which they talk about and experience emotions. For example, expressions of anger may be avoided in some cultures and may even shape the way in which individuals experience the feeling of anger. In this book we will focus on both how grownups can better understand their child's individual response and how grownups can respond when children are dysregulated.

When children reach their preschool years they begin to separate from their grownups more, needing to manage their emotions more autonomously as a result. What is commonly referred to as temper tantrums decrease as they approach the preschool years (Van den Akker, Hoffenaar and Overbeek 2022). Developmentally, the significant growth in communication skills which occurs around this time supports this shift. Siegel (2020) suggests that early patterns of co-regulation are likely to shape the way in which children manage emotions at this age and stage. For example, research has demonstrated that securely attached children were more likely to seek the support of a teacher to co-regulate, whereas those with avoidant attachment patterns were less likely to do so (Stefan and Negrean 2021). More generally the literature indicates that interactions between parents and children influence emotion processing and regulation neurocircuitry, which in turn impacts on a child's mental health and wellbeing (Tan *et al.* 2020).

The neuroscience of regulation

As a therapist, rather than a neuroscientist, my understanding of the brain is simplistic. Knowledge of neuroscience and interpersonal neurobiology has increased markedly in recent years, and it has become clear that, while we as therapists may lack a technical and detailed understanding, we must integrate these learnings into our practice. In this section I will explore some of the key learnings that are emerging, conveying these simply and exploring what this means for therapy. These points are drawn from Siegel (2020) and I would urge interested readers to read his books for themselves.

Children (and grownups) have what Siegel (2020) terms a "window of tolerance." This is the amount of emotional arousal that we can process before our system is unable to function. The size of our window varies and can be influenced by our experiences. For example, children who are encouraged to take appropriate risks in play may be less likely to become dysregulated by new challenges. On the other hand, children who have been repeatedly frightened and have not had the support of a soothing grownup may have a very narrow window of tolerance. Internal and external conditions alter the size of our window in any given moment. For example, hunger and fatigue may make our window smaller and make us more prone to becoming dysregulated. This book includes some ideas about how you can explore this with children and families and includes some ideas about how you can stay within your own window of tolerance.

Moving beyond our window of tolerance (or becoming dysregulated) leads to disruptions in our thinking and behavior. Many children engage in behavior when angry that is impulsive and reckless, and it is important to understand that they are not using their higher cognitive functions, such as problem-solving and reflection, when they are in this state. When emotionally flooded in this way children (and grownups) find themselves reacting impulsively without thinking. It is also helpful for grownups to understand that the child may move into having a freeze or flight response at this time, or as is frequently observed with children who present with anger issues, a fight reaction.

Our knowledge of regulation also needs to shape the way in which we work with children. One implication is that we need to regulate children before we can ask them to use their thinking skills, calming their bodies first. Our higher brain structures, those that allow for social engagement and for creative thought, are only accessible when we feel safe. In order to help children learn to be able to make good choices when they are angry, we need to return them to their window of tolerance, to a space in which they can notice how they are feeling, while still being able to think about the situation and mindfully choose how they wish to respond. It is essential that we reflect this in our therapy, emphasizing the need for regulation and only engaging in higher-level cognitive processes when a child is regulated.

It is also important to acknowledge that conscious processes, such as problem-solving and cognitive strategies, develop throughout childhood and adolescence. While a child's developmental level is clearly influential here, with younger children being less able to use conscious processes such as problem-solving or cognitive strategies, the child's individual experience is also crucial. The children I see tend to become quickly dysregulated and have little access to conscious processes when they do so. They often have not had an experience of being effectively co-regulated. In this context we often begin with helping the grownups to create a more supportive environment for them and co-regulate with them while we begin helping the child to tune in more to their body and early warning signs that they are becoming dysregulated. Chapter 2 helps you to reflect on what you learn from your early sessions with a child and to begin thinking about what they need therapeutically.

We also know that emotions themselves are regulating. As Siegel (2020) eloquently puts this, "emotion and emotion regulation are seen as woven from the same cloth" (p.232), such that emotions are regulated in addition to providing a regulating function. The first part of this statement reflects the need to regulate emotions, and for this reason, you will see a focus on regulation throughout this book, along with activities specifically addressing this process early in the book. The latter idea, namely that emotions also provide regulation, is also adopted in these pages. So often the experience of expressing our feelings and having them acknowledged is, in and of itself, regulating. This is why you will see an emphasis on exploring a child's anger and validating their feelings.

Siegel (2020) also points to the role of consciousness, noting that having awareness allows us to make a choice to do something differently. When we are aware of our feelings and typical reactions in the moment as well as our patterns of responding over time, we are more alert to this and can intentionally make a choice to do something differently. As children develop what is referred to as metacognition, they are able to think about their thoughts, form a representation of their own mind, be aware of their own self-beliefs and understand the nature of emotion. For this reason, our early sessions focus on helping children and their grownups to understand some of the patterns that are occurring and become more conscious of these. Chapter 5 focuses on helping children and families understand anger.

Neuroscience also helps us understand why change takes time. Neural pathways strengthen the more they are used, enabling increasingly automatic ways of responding. While this is helpful in some areas, it can be unhelpful in others. Both children and grownups can have strong, automatic responses in response to particular triggers or internal experiences. For example, the child who has repeatedly felt ashamed in the context of not knowing how to complete her schoolwork may feel unsafe when faced with not knowing in other contexts, which may trigger a fight or flight response. Changing these patterns requires a consciousness about the experience and an active choice to respond differently, developing a new neural pathway over time. We'll talk more about this later in this chapter.

Regulation and the therapeutic relationship

Perhaps most importantly, we know that the therapeutic relationship is incredibly important and our interactions with the child and family can help them to feel safe. Polyvagal theory emphasizes the role of social engagement in creating safety (Porges 2017). While therapists are generally very aware of our non-verbal responses in sessions and of building a supportive therapeutic relationship, Porges' theory has helped us to understand why having vocal prosody, a warm and welcoming facial expression and gestures of accessibility are so valuable. Our neural circuits use a neural process, which Porges terms *neuroception,* to identify whether situations are safe or unsafe. This process, which occurs at an unconscious level, can help children and grownups feel safe in the therapy space. Treisman (2017) notes that children who have experienced relational and developmental trauma are particularly attuned to, and may misinterpret, signals of threat, meaning that we need to be particularly mindful of creating safety in this context.

Safety is likely to look slightly different to each person; however, Treisman (2017) highlights the need for multi-leveled safety, encompassing inner safety, emotional safety, physical safety and felt safety. Dion (2018) further suggests that physical threat, as well as the unknown and incongruence, are perceived as threats, creating a sense that situations are unsafe. Having unrealistic expectations is also described as a threat (Dion 2018). Safety is a prerequisite for all therapeutic work and needs to be prioritized throughout our work with children and families.

Interpersonal neurobiology is helping us understand the way in which we impact, and are impacted by, others. The therapeutic relationship is an example of this, with dynamic and bidirectional communication between bodily states and emotions as the therapist and client interact (Porges 2017). The nature of this communication highlights the need for therapists to be aware of their own feelings and emotions, both in sessions and more generally. Therapists need to be able to tune in to their feelings and regulate themselves in order to effectively support children and families. Throughout this book you will see some prompts that encourage you to reflect on your own experience of anger and how you can keep yourself regulated in sessions, with the understanding that doing so protects the therapeutic relationship.

Anger and diagnosis

One of the challenges of identifying the prevalence of anger difficulties is that these can vary in presentation. To date, much of the research has focused on diagnostic categories, such as oppositional defiant disorder (ODD) or attention deficit hyperactivity disorder (ADHD). Even when researchers have avoided diagnostic categories, they have relied on different descriptions, using terms like aggression, irritability and tantrums.

Between 2019 and 2021 the American Academy of Child and Adolescent Psychiatry Presidential Task Force conducted a narrative review on impairing emotional outbursts independent of diagnosis. Noting the limitations of the available research, the task force estimated that emotionally impairing outbursts occur in 4–10% of children in the community, from preschoolers to adolescents (Carlson *et al.* 2023).

Many of these children present to mental health professionals, accounting for a significant proportion of all referrals. For example, Smith and colleagues (2018) found that of referrals to Child and Adolescent Mental Health Services (CAMHS) in Scotland just under one third were for emotional and behavioral problems. More generally, Carlson *et al.* (2023) found that outbursts in children were responsible for significant numbers of referrals to emergency departments, inpatient units, schools, outpatient clinics and residential treatment settings.

Sometimes children are diagnosed with a disorder in which anger and behavior difficulties are a key feature. This includes ODD, conduct disorder and the more recent disruptive mood regulation disorder (American Psychiatric Association 2013). Importantly however, anger and emotional dysregulation are also commonly seen in a broad range of childhood psychiatric difficulties, including in children with anxiety and mood difficulties, in neurodiverse children and in children who have experienced trauma (Carlson *et al.* 2023). Diagnosis can be helpful and addressing underlying disorders can help reduce angry outbursts. For example, children with ADHD who are effectively managed on stimulant medication may be less likely to respond impulsively, which can reduce angry outbursts.

Diagnosis is, however, only part of the picture. In practice many children present with more than one disorder or don't fit neatly into our diagnostic categories. Furthermore, children who have the same diagnosis can present very differently and have different clinical trajectories. Indeed, a number of studies have identified subtypes of children with ODD (e.g., Wesselhoeft *et al.* 2019). More broadly, a recent person-centered longitudinal study exploring internalizing, externalizing and peer difficulties across childhood identified a number of different trajectories, with difficulties in one domain being associated with difficulties in the other domains (Girard 2021).

A diagnosis, therefore, provides us with a picture of a child's current difficulties, though it may provide little insight as to how these difficulties came to be and what other challenges the child might be experiencing. Further, attributing angry outbursts to a disorder can prevent us from exploring the function of the behavior or exploring what it might be communicating (Carlson *et al.* 2023). Focusing on an individual child's symptoms and understanding the context around these enables us to provide targeted intervention. The research of Thöne *et al.* (2023) highlights the need to consider the functional impact of individual symptoms, suggesting that doing so is often useful in planning intervention.

This book is written for therapists who work with children who find it hard to regulate and manage their anger, regardless of their diagnosis or presentation. Individual assessment that leads to a thorough understanding of a child's challenges within the context of their early experiences and family life is crucial. Such an understanding may include a diagnosis; however, it is far deeper. Achieving this level of understanding can only occur in the context of a safe and secure therapeutic relationship. Chapter 2 helps guide your assessment of the child and family, supporting you to collaboratively develop a shared understanding of the challenges prior to moving into therapy.

Theoretical frameworks and evidence base

Throughout this book you will find playful strategies for use with children in therapy. A play-based approach is a natural fit when working with children, aligning with their developmental needs. Play is in and of itself naturally regulating, allowing the child to remain connected while they explore and learn. Furthermore, play is active, allowing the child to do, rather than say, and more effectively bridging the space between the child's day-to-day life and therapy. In *The Therapeutic Powers of Play*, Schaefer and Drewes (2014) describe the ways in which play is inherently powerful and can lead to behavior change. Later in this book you will see activities that draw on many of these therapeutic powers of play, including self-expression, stress management, and direct and indirect teaching.

Most of the activities in this book utilize play in a directive manner, allowing the child to explore their anger or have a different experience of their anger. Many of these activities were created as I worked with children. Often I was following their lead and saw an opportunity to become more directive and introduce a therapeutic concept, with these activities emerging as part of the process. This allowed me to introduce the activity with other children at relevant points in therapy. The activities included in this book therefore are directive and conscious, fitting primarily within Quadrant II of Yasenik and Gardner's (2012) model for those of you who are familiar with this. The activities provide an opportunity to use play to introduce and allow children to explore therapeutic concepts. Many of the activities are based on the newer cognitive behavioral therapies, acceptance and commitment therapy (ACT) and dialectical behavior therapy (DBT). There are also influences of narrative therapy and emotion-focused therapy. Each activity is play-based, ensuring it is developmentally appropriate and there is a focus on working with the family throughout.

Note: All activities and handouts marked with a ✳ can be photocopied or downloaded from www.jkp.com/catalogue/book/9781839975561

In terms of an evidence base, therefore, the approach in this book draws on findings from a number of areas. There is good evidence for the use of CBT in children with anger difficulties (e.g., Lachman *et al.* 2021). In addition there is some research supporting the use of DBT and ACT in children with emotional regulation difficulties (Berkout, Tinsley and Flynn 2020; Perepletchikova *et al.* 2017), although further research is needed. There is also research to suggest that these approaches can be helpful with children with autism (e.g., Clifford *et al.* 2022). Parenting work, often referred to as parent-management training, is also considered a key component of managing anger and aggression difficulties in children and has a good evidence base (Kazdin 2017). Carlson *et al.* (2023) note that most of the evidence-based approaches for angry outbursts are founded on the principles of behavior modification and cognitive behavior therapy, including CBT, ACT, DBT and parent-management training, as is the approach outlined in this book. The clinical approach of this book is also grounded in our understanding of the neuroscience of regulation and in developmental theory. The latter is exemplified in the playful approach we undertake throughout as well as the inclusion of family in therapy. Developmental considerations are described in each of the sections, allowing you to adapt your approach according to the age and stage of the child.

One advantage of drawing on a range of therapeutic approaches is that it provides flexibility for the therapist to meet the needs of the individual child and family. Indeed, Carlson *et al.* (2023) advocate for therapists needing a "tool belt of effective therapies that can be mixed and matched to address the specific needs of a child and family" (p.141). The activities in this book are intended to be used according to your clinical judgment, rather than in a prescribed order. Some children and families will need more support to understand anger, while others will need greater time focusing on developing calming and coping strategies. Some will need to spend more time on co-regulation, while others will benefit most from cognitive strategies. Tracking the progress of therapy in an ongoing way is essential, enabling us to know whether our therapeutic approach is working and adjust it if need be. This approach is discussed further in Chapter 3.

On language

Throughout this book, I have used the term *child* to refer to the client, though please feel free to adopt the language that suits best for you. The activities included are generally appropriate for children aged between 4 and 12 years though you are encouraged to use your clinical judgment to identify which activities are appropriate for the children you see. In this book I have referred to younger and older children when describing therapeutic activities and practical suggestions for working with children and families. When I say older children, I am generally referring to those over 8 or so years of age, with the understanding that children tend to be more able to reflect on their thoughts by this age and engage in more complex problem-solving. Younger children, those under 8 or so, tend to need more hands-on strategies and greater support from grownups. This is a broad division of what is, in reality, a continuum, with younger children needing more support and cognitive abilities becoming better developed over time. There are also, of course, significant differences in the ages at which children develop, and I would encourage you to consider the developmental age of the children you see, so do consider the individual child you are working with and adapt accordingly.

I have used the term *neurodiversity* to refer to conditions such as autism and ADHD, noting those conditions specifically when relevant. I have used both identity-first and person-first language throughout, with the understanding that different children and families prefer different terms here. I encourage you to check in with individual families around this and to remain aware of the changes in this space, knowing that at some point in the future these will likely date the language I have used here.

I have used the term *family* throughout to identify those the child lives with, regardless of the configuration this takes. Similarly, I have used the term *grownups* for a child's carers, regardless of whether they are the child's biological family. The emphasis on involving grownups and family throughout reflects the need to work with the child's system, for it is only when we do so that we can create substantial and long-lasting change.

Throughout the book, you will see short vignettes, which provide an illustration of what is being discussed. These are not case examples, though they have been created from compilations of children and families I have seen over the years. Details have been changed and merged in order to ensure that confidentiality is protected.

Knowing your own feelings about anger

JASMINE

During supervision, Jasmine wanted to discuss a 9-year-old child who had been referred for angry outbursts. As the discussion progressed, it became clear that the 9-year-old was expressing appropriate anger toward his older brother; however, his mother, whose own early experiences of anger had felt unpredictable and scary, was finding this very challenging. As she worked through this, Jasmine realized that her own beliefs about anger and her tendency to repress her own anger had caused her to accept the mother's narrative around her son's behavior. She began to reflect on how she might create an opportunity to hear what the boy was trying to communicate through his anger, supporting the family to understand that his expression of anger was developmentally appropriate.

Having good self-awareness is important for therapists (Miller and Moyers 2021), particularly given the importance of the therapeutic relationship as discussed previously. It is essential, therefore, that we explore our own relationship with anger. Our own experiences of anger, our emotional responses when anger arises and our focus on content in therapy can all make it difficult to manage anger within sessions.

It is inevitable that our own feelings and thoughts arise in our work with children and families. This is part of the process of therapy and can, indeed, be helpful at times. What is key, however, is that we have a good awareness of how our own experiences have shaped our responses and know what is likely to come up for us in therapy. Consciously reflecting on our own experience of anger, both growing up and in the present, can elicit some new understandings of how we approach this emotion. Our feelings about the feeling, which Gottman, Katz and Hooven (1996) termed *meta-emotion*, are essential to understand if we are to really appreciate why we might respond the way we do in the moment to expressions of anger. Take some time to explore this for yourself using the prompts in the box below. Sharing some of your reflections with your supervisor is also likely to help, so too journaling and reflecting with colleagues and loved ones. Individual therapy can be helpful as well, particularly if you've had traumatic experiences of anger.

Questions to ask yourself about anger

Was anger safe or unsafe?

Was it unpredictable or fitting with the context?

Was it appropriately expressed or was it chaotic and scary?

What were some of the messages I received about anger?

What feelings come up for me when others express anger?

What are the bodily sensations I notice when others are angry?

How do I respond to others being angry?

What are my thoughts and beliefs around anger?

How do I express my own anger?

How do I respond when I am angry?

What do I notice in my body?

How do I typically express my anger?

Having a good awareness of our own relationship with anger enables us to know how we are likely to respond to others expressing anger in the clinic room. Our responses to anger convey a lot about our attitudes toward anger in addition to offering an opportunity for modeling regulation and appropriate expression. For example, if we are able to regulate a child through their anger and get curious about this feeling, we offer the child a very different experience to one in which we become anxious in response to their anger and set limits without empathizing or offering regulation strategies. Being aware of our typical responses prompts us to regulate ourselves and supports us to respond in a more mindful manner.

Sometimes the emotions that are elicited in response to anger arising in the room relate to the context of therapy. Thoughts such as "I'm incompetent," "This is not working," "I have to get to that activity" or "I haven't even had a chance to talk about…" can trigger feelings of hopelessness or anxiety. When therapists experience these thoughts and feelings, they often become dysregulated themselves and, as a result, become less attuned and less able to regulate the child and/or grownups. If a child becomes angry in a session, this can feel like an added stress, something else that needs to be sorted in your short time with a child and family. However, when we embrace the moment and see helping the child and family to regulate through these feelings as an important part of our work, we provide something very powerful indeed.

Reflection and self-awareness is an ongoing process. Structures such as supervision can help facilitate this, and it is essential to consider how you can promote reflective practice for yourself in an ongoing way.

Regulation for therapists

I'm taking a big breath as I walk to greet the family in my waiting room, knowing there is a lot going on for them and that they often bring a lot of anxiety in the form of anger into the room. During the session I take sips from my water bottle as needed and move a little to help me stay regulated. I name their feelings and label my own, saying that it all feels a bit overwhelming and wondering if this is part of what they are feeling too. I suggest that we all pause and take a breath on a few occasions and at one point we decide to take a five-minute break. The grownups make a cup of tea while the child plays and everyone returns to the session more regulated.

How we feel in the room impacts on the way we interact with the child and their family, so it is essential that we are aware of this. If we are feeling uncomfortable and don't express this, the family will often pick up on it, noticing the incongruence. Being dysregulated also impacts on our ability to be present with the child and family and makes it difficult for us to regulate them when we need to. Having an awareness of our feelings is an important first step toward regulation. Awareness does not prevent us from becoming dysregulated; however, it does prepare us for the likelihood that this will happen and helps us predict when this might happen. Having an awareness of our own responses also helps us to make sense of what is happening when we do become dysregulated, and it supports us to regulate, connecting to ourselves and owning the experience.

As with children, one of the first steps in regulation is to notice our own feelings and to name them. Being able to tune in and notice our feelings often provides useful information. Sometimes the feelings that arise in us give us valuable information about the experience of the child or their grownups, so being able to name what we are feeling for ourselves is clinically helpful. Other times, what we are feeling relates more to our own experiences, and reflecting on this supports our own development. Sometimes naming these feelings out loud with the family, as in the example above, can be very helpful. This can highlight an aspect of their experience that they were not tuning in to and often facilitates further discussion.

In addition to naming, you can regulate yourself in the session, using strategies such as breathing, taking a drink and moving your body, again as in the example above. This allows the child and grownups to indirectly learn about regulation and to see it in action. Another useful aspect of these strategies is that they tend to slow the session, allowing everyone to pause for a moment, which is often regulating in and of itself.

Beyond how you regulate yourself in sessions, it is worth thinking about what you do between sessions that helps you to stay regulated. Scheduling your sessions in a way that works well for you is important, and when doing so it is worth thinking about what helps you to stay regulated both between sessions and across the day. More generally, having a rhythm to your year, with regular breaks, and surrounding yourself with good support will help you stay regulated.

The role of play and using playful activities

The playful activities included throughout this book are categorized according to whether they are helpful for first sessions, for supporting children to understand anger, for developing calming strategies or for thinking about anger. These activities are essentially a child-friendly way of introducing a therapeutic concept, providing a way of helping children to understand and explore these. Given this, it is therefore essential that the activities are integrated into practice. Indeed, it is the conversations we have around activities that are often the most important. Implicit in this is the idea of repetition. Through repetition the therapeutic concepts become more meaningful to the child and more relatable to their day-to-day life. For this reason, you will also see that many of the activities touch on the same concept, providing repetition and extension.

Rather than being presented as a standardized therapy program, the activities in this book are designed to be chosen according to the individual needs of the child and family you are working with. Therefore, you need to be able to assess in an ongoing way, have a good understanding of the child and family's challenges and be guided by your therapeutic goals, choosing activities that fit within this framework. It can be tempting to use therapeutic activities much in the way you would a recipe, running through these in a methodical way. Therapy is, however, so much more than this, and it is essential that you bring your knowledge of the individual child and family to each of the activities, adapting and modifying these to meet their needs. How you present an activity should be shaped very much by your understanding of how the child experiences anger, linking the activity with concepts you have covered previously, and considering carefully how the family might be able to incorporate the learning into their day-to-day life. Most of the activities offer a couple of different ways to present the idea, so think about what option might be best for the children you work with. Reflect on aspects such as whether or not they need movement in the session, think about the language they use and incorporate that into the activity, and ensure that you present it in a way that fits with their developmental level. It is also helpful to ensure that the child is regulated prior to introducing an activity.

The activities often provide an opportunity for you to share some of your own feelings, allowing you to draw on the therapeutic power of indirect teaching while also normalizing the child's experience. Giving of yourself in this way is also playful and can support engagement. Obviously, whatever you share needs to be appropriate, meeting the child's needs rather than your own. Sharing day-to-day examples is often the best place to start, such as being worried and angry when your train was canceled and you were late to work. Throughout the activities, I have suggested that you engage a child's grownups similarly.

Importantly, it is essential that we stay present when using therapeutic activities. Sometimes, because these activities elicit communication between children and their grownups, there can be a tendency to focus on what is said rather than on what is happening in the moment. We need to be attuned to the child throughout the activity, being curious about their experience of the activity. For example, a child who talks comfortably about feeling happy though has nothing to say about anger is conveying a discomfort with this feeling. Similarly, a child who sits with their head down and talks about how they sometimes do the wrong thing by hitting out at others may be communicating the shame they experience about their anger, as well as a tendency to internalize what grownups have said about their behavior.

If a child becomes dysregulated during an activity, expressing anger or even becoming overly excited, pausing and working through this by regulating them is essential. At a basic level this might be about simplifying our explanation in response to noticing that a child looks confused. It may also be about slowing our pace when a child is reluctant to share examples of times when they feel angry and moving to simply offering examples of when you feel angry or asking about what might make their friends angry. At a more complex level it might be about noticing that something about the language you have used has been triggering for the child or grownup and regulating them through this so that you can explore this together once everyone has returned to a state of regulation. Ensuring that you are regulated places you in a good position to monitor the child's and family's reactions closely throughout, watching for early signs of dysregulation so that you can pause sooner rather than later and offer some bottom-up calming strategies. This might be about taking a break, moving your body or getting a drink.

One implication of this is that we need to allow time to complete activities. Pace is essential, and normally, as a guide, I would recommend doing one activity in a session. This allows for you and the child to immerse yourselves in the activity, enables you to draw connections with previous sessions and to thoughtfully reflect on how the child and family can use this learning between this session and the next. Obviously, pace also needs to be considered in the context of the individual child and their learning rate too, with some children requiring a greater amount of repetition.

Allowing time to reflect on an activity is also important. Talking about how the child found the activity and what they noticed during the activity is often useful. Starting with general reflections, such as "I wonder what your thoughts about that game are" or "I'd be interested to hear what that was like for you," often works well. Suggested reflections are included in each activity write-up. Ideally, it is useful to focus the reflections both on what the child and family have learnt from an activity and how this understanding might be utilized outside of sessions. You can also share what you noticed and invite the child to share their thoughts about this. Reflection is also an opportunity to further link the activity with what you have previously covered in therapy. For example, you might say something like "We've been talking a lot about those worry thoughts, and I know you noticed some as we were playing that game today. Did you have those thoughts the whole time we were playing?"

What you reflect on will vary depending on the child's experience of the task and where you are at in the therapy process overall. It can be tempting to highlight the learning in an activity; however, exploring the child's experience and taking whatever they have learnt from the task is preferable. This also helps us to get a sense of where they are at and what they might need. It is also important that this reflection does not continue for too long. Engaging in too much discussion leads to children disengaging. Similarly, there may be aspects of the task that you choose to reflect on later with the grownups rather than explore further with the child. Again, this comes down to your clinical judgment. A final, though important, part of reflection involves thinking about how the family might use activity or the learning that has come from it at home. This grounds the work you have been doing and supports the family to integrate this into their day-to-day life. It also supports the grownups to see the relevance of what you are doing in sessions.

All of the above points also relate to working online with children and families, and most of the activities include a suggestion for how this could be used online. Online work has some additional challenges, so if you are working in this manner please also read the section in Chapter 9 on this.

The importance of grownups

The value of having a supportive relationship with an attuned adult cannot be overstated, and it is helpful to understand who might play this role for a child prior to commencing therapy. Even weekly therapy is a small amount of time in a child's life, and, as therapists, we need to be realistic about what we can achieve in this time. Being able to work with at least one supportive grownup helps us to ensure that the child can be supported in their day-to-day life, knowing that what we can achieve is greatly magnified when we can work closely with the child's grownups. Much in the way that safety is the basis for our therapeutic relationship with children, we also need to remember that the relationships a child experiences outside of therapy create safety, which is essential if they are to be well supported.

By the time children come to therapy, their relationship with their grownups is often strained. Many have had longstanding challenges and have not experienced an attuned relationship with their grownups. Throughout therapy, therefore, we need to work closely with children and their grownups, working to foster understanding and build connection. Some of the activities, such as animal shapes in Chapter 4, have a strong focus on connection; however, even when that is not the case, each activity provides an opportunity for communication and for building understanding and empathy. Supporting children and grownups to engage more effectively throughout these activities is a priority.

Supporting the relationship between a child and their grownups requires time. Quickly moving through content often detracts from this, meaning that we miss important opportunities in which we might otherwise have helped a grownup connect with their child, sharing moments of enjoyment and understanding. So slow down, reflect on your own stance in the therapy room, and capture those moments rather than moving through activities too quickly. Regulate children and grownups as needed and provide time for them to explore what is happening between them, particularly when there are examples of attunement or misattunement.

Generally the activities will suggest that both you and the child's grownups engage actively in the activities. Helping grownups to do so requires us to orient them to the process, support them to know what is and isn't appropriate and help them to navigate this even when big feelings arise in the room. Importantly, grownups need to feel safe in order to be able to share of themselves in this way, and the relationship we need to establish with them is similar to that which we create for the child. Being clear, right from your initial contact with the family, about what your expectations are around grownups being in the room and being actively involved is helpful. Creating a space in which grownups can explore their feelings about this is essential, as is talking together about what grownups might be able to share in the room. Even with the best preparation however, grownups can sometimes become dysregulated in sessions. As with children, we need to closely watch and support them throughout, providing opportunities for regulation as needed to enable them to be present for their child. The box below outlines some helpful suggestions on having grownups actively involved in therapy.

Helping grownups engage actively in therapy

Be clear about the expectation from the outset.

Explore grownups' feelings about being involved.

Provide information about how sessions will work.

Include examples of what grownups might share in sessions.

Identify how you can support grownups through sessions.

Encourage grownups to seek your support as needed.

Actively monitor grownups throughout the session.

Provide regulation as needed.

By involving grownups and families right from the start, we send a clear message that grownups are important. This can be challenging for grownups who assume they are not part of the problem and simply want their child "fixed," and there is often some work around helping the family to see the connections. On the other hand, though, involving grownups and families clearly positions them as part of the solution. It privileges their perspectives and empowers them, creating change that continues long after therapy ends. The active engagement of grownups also allows us to increase the intensity of the work we are doing, allowing the grownup to respond therapeutically in the child's day-to-day life, rather than limiting therapy to the confines of our sessions. Furthermore, involving grownups allows for children to be supported in the moment, as they experience the emotions, and to explore other ways of responding. This perhaps is where the true power of involving grownups lies; in the ability to respond in the moment and in doing so creating a different experience, one which is far more based in the body than any subsequent discussion of that experience will be in the clinic room.

The above points are, I believe, true for all of our work with children. It is valuable, though, to take a few moments and consider these points as they relate specifically to anger. Most children who are referred for difficulties with anger will have difficulty managing their emotions in a range of environments, including at home. These children need support to regulate, which can be difficult for grownups. Most of us, as therapists, have had the experience of being a co-regulator within our sessions. We notice signs that a child is becoming heightened and connect with our own feelings in the moment, connecting to our experience so that we can provide them an experience of regulation. Many of us feel very comfortable in this role and do it effortlessly, and there is undoubtedly a benefit to the child to have this experience of being regulated. Consider, though, how much more powerful it would be to support the grownup to regulate their child.

When we help grownups to be more regulated, we create a calmer home environment for the child; however, more importantly, we also create in the grownup a co-regulator who is far more available than us. We create a co-regulator who can be there for a child more often when the child is angry, whether that is when they are in the car on the way home from school or as they are playing soccer after school with their siblings. Having grownups who can regulate their children means that children get more practice of working through their anger. The sheer number of times that a grownup is likely to be available to co-regulate their child is likely to be far greater, allowing for more opportunities and greater repetition and for more efficient learning.

Further, grownups are much more likely to be available to regulate their child in their day-to-day life, which makes this experience all the more powerful. Most of us as therapists have had the experience of talking with a child and their grownups about a time they got angry after the fact, noting that they could reflect thoughtfully about what they could have done differently. The space in which children and their grownups talk calmly about something that has happened in the past is quite different to the experience of a child in the moment. Sitting and reflecting after the fact is often a more cognitive space and, for grownups, often quite different to having a supported experience in the moment of regulating the child. We'll talk more about how to facilitate this regulation process throughout the book.

In addition to co-regulation, grownups are also well placed to support their child in other ways. Attuned grownups are able to readily gauge their child's level of regulation, building calming rhythms into their day as needed. They understand their child's triggers and pace their expectations, allowing them to prepare for and gradually face challenging situations. Their awareness of their child's needs as well as their strengths allows them to create a supportive environment that allows for an appropriate mix of support and challenge.

More generally, the way a family interacts around anger shapes a child's experience of this. Children might learn that anger is an important emotion, one that prompts important communication, or they may form the belief that anger is to be avoided and suppressed. They may learn that anger is something that is unsafe and scary, or that anger can be expressed appropriately and can be followed by repair.

Grownups therefore need to be closely involved in therapy. They are a necessary part of the co-regulation process; a crucial piece of the therapy puzzle for children who are yet to develop this skill. They are more able to be present in those settings when the child needs support to regulate and, when well supported, can continue supporting the child long after therapy is finished.

Finding new paths

There is a path I am fortunate enough to walk often: a beautiful wide path that leads to a beach I love. Paved and direct, it can be traveled quickly, and I am convinced that you could put me on it blindfolded and I would still travel it safely. Having walked this path so many times allows me to do so automatically and quickly, without thought or hesitation.

Some time ago I had the pleasure of walking another path to a different beach, one that leads from a friend's house to a remote ocean beach. The track is a narrow dirt one and was quite overgrown at the time, having not been used for some months. I felt excited, though uncertain, as I walked the path, reassured to be following my friend, and moving slowly and cautiously.

I've shared this story about the two different paths many times with families and colleagues as it reminds me very much of the process of therapy. We all have ways of responding to situations that are automatic and fast, paths that we travel often in response to situations, events and emotions. We travel these paths automatically and efficiently, without pausing to consider or think about what we are doing. The way we respond in times of emotion is no different. Many of the children we work with respond automatically with anger in times of anxiety or disappointment, treading a well-worn path. Similarly, their grownups will respond in their own often-traveled way, which may date back to their own childhood.

The more we engage in a behavioral response the more we will tend to do so. This is because our neural pathways work to become efficient and automatic. And so the pathways described above can be considered a metaphor for our neural pathways, allowing us to consider our automatic responses and reflect on what it means to respond in a different way.

What this means, first and foremost, is that children and their grownups are often unaware of the paths they travel when angry. Learning about anger, looking for the feelings underneath, and becoming curious about patterns can help children and grownups to understand their responses and become more aware of the path they are walking. As noted previously, it is this conscious awareness that allows us to choose to respond differently. For most grownups, tracing the origins of their path back to their childhood can be really helpful, so opening up a space in which they can explore their own early experiences of anger is encouraged.

The automatic nature of emotional responses means that changing behaviors that have become automatic is difficult and slow. Paths can only become well-traveled over time. The overgrown path I traveled with my friend that day would have been clearer and wider by the end of summer as a result of being walked. Neural pathways are no different. To engage in a new way of responding requires conscious thought and effort. It is time-consuming and inefficient and can only become automatic after much practice. What this means is that for the children and grownups we work with (and indeed for ourselves) we need to recognize that change will take time. We need to provide lots of empathy around this and encourage children and grownups to be kind to themselves as they develop new paths.

The friend who led me down the new path that day took the role of a guide. As therapists, we are often in the position of guiding children and grownups along a new path. Our presence, much in the way I experienced the presence of my friend that day, is valuable and supportive. It is far easier to walk a new path with support than to do it alone, particularly initially. I often reflect on this when I think about the process of therapy and the need to create experiences within sessions that allow children and grownups to try a new way of responding. The activities in this book often bring some emotion into the room, allowing you to support both children and grownups to respond differently, rather than reacting in the way they typically would. In doing so you help guide them down a different path.

The final aspect of this metaphor that I tend to explore with grownups is that each time we walk a path we make it easier to travel again. Walking a path widens and flattens it; walking it increases our knowledge of the path and, in turn, increases our ability to travel the path more effectively. What this means in practice is that each time we manage to do something different we are beginning to alter our behavior; we are working toward creating a new path. Remembering this allows me to express curiosity and amazement whenever a child or a grownup is able to respond differently when angry, reminding them that it will become easier each time they do so. It creates space for grownups to understand that it will take time for children to learn a new way and recognize the role they play in supporting this. It also allows us to hold with kindness all of the moments when grownups react to their child's anger in the same old way, having empathy for how readily we follow our well-traveled paths and reassurance that new paths can be developed over time.

Most grownups readily understand this metaphor, and it is one we return to again and again, noticing when they or their child have managed to walk a different path. Sometimes I will use this with older children too, drawing a line on a page to show the child that the path becomes wider and quicker to draw the more we do it.

The metaphor is one that is useful for us as therapists too. The approach presented in this book may be a new one for you and you may find yourself returning to the way you previously worked despite wanting to try something new. Trying to be mindful of this and giving yourself the time to consciously walk a new path, knowing that doing so can be difficult, is helpful. Enjoy the journey.

CHAPTER 2

FIRST SESSIONS

This chapter explores some considerations for your first sessions with children and their families, along with some playful assessment activities. These first sessions allow us to begin building a relationship with the child and their grownups and help them to understand what coming to therapy might involve. We learn a lot about the family, both from what they say and what we observe. Ideally, too, these initial sessions are therapeutic for the child and their grownups. The telling of their story may be healing in and of itself, and a skilled therapist will facilitate moments of connection and different ways of understanding in the first sessions, supporting therapeutic growth.

First sessions with a child and their grownups will look different for each family. The child's developmental level, the family makeup and dynamics and the way in which children and their grownups engage with the process should shape content, format and pace of your first sessions. Your theoretical orientation and the setting in which you work will also undoubtedly influence the way in which you structure your first sessions; however, it is your clinical skills and your engagement with the family that will ultimately make first sessions helpful for the child and their grownups. With that in mind, this chapter offers some suggestions around how to approach the assessment space and what to cover.

It is important to note that I am referring to first sessions, knowing that you may have one or two initial assessment sessions or as many as six depending on the context in which you work. Further, the boundary between assessment and therapy is an artificial one: assessment remains important throughout therapy and therapy begins from our first moments with the family. Some children and their grownups will readily present their story, providing a clear picture within the first session, while others will gradually share more information over time.

Finding the balance

Effective therapy is embedded in thorough assessment. It is our understanding of the child and family that allows us to choose appropriate interventions, ensuring that you pace these appropriately. Although difficulties with anger have often been identified at the point of referral, it is essential that we undertake our own assessment. The process of assessment facilitates not only our own understanding, it also supports the child and family to develop an understanding too. It forges a partnership between the child and family and the therapist, and lays a foundation for the therapy work that is to follow.

One of the challenges in first sessions is finding the balance between collecting assessment information, building rapport and orientating the child and family to the therapy process. As therapists, we often see the focus of the initial assessment session as involving the collection of information; however, if we don't focus on building a relationship with the child and family, the information we collect is irrelevant. Children and grownups who don't feel secure with the therapist in the first session are unlikely to return to therapy, which means that the assessment information collected will remain unused. Further, children and grownups who don't feel safe within the therapeutic relationship are unlikely to provide accurate assessment information. Consider for example, the child who feels unsure of the therapist and shares only a little of their experience of anger, or the parent who feels defensive and tells the therapist how they would like to respond to their child's anger rather than how they actually do respond.

It takes time to build a relationship, and there inevitably will be a deepening over time that enables the child and family to share more of their experience. With some families, this process takes longer; with others, it is shorter. Families who have little experience of positive relationships, have a history of trauma and negative interactions with services will likely need us to focus more on the therapeutic relationship. Taking the time to focus on the relationship early in the process, however, and pacing our information gathering to suit the child and family, all helps to provide a strong basis for therapeutic work.

Helping children and families to understand the process of therapy is also important in our first sessions. All too often, we forget that the family may not have engaged in therapy before. Indeed, even when the family has a prior experience of therapy, it may be very different to what you provide within the context of your setting. It is essential, therefore, that in the assessment phase we are helping the child and family to understand what they can expect. This is important both at a session level, as well as more broadly. Early sessions should begin with the therapist explaining what will happen in the session and ensuring the child and family have understood this. In addition the broader process of therapy should be outlined, including what working with the therapist will entail, how sessions will look, who will be involved, how you will develop and review goals, and how they can raise concerns. Obviously, there are aspects of this process that will be unknown, such as how long therapy might continue for or what the content of sessions will be; however, explaining this to the family helps them to know that you will communicate with them through the process, explaining your thinking, exploring theirs and working collaboratively. Engaging in this manner often decreases the family's anxiety and supports their engagement, both with the therapist and with the process of therapy.

First sessions with children
Setting up the space for children

ZANE

Zane's mother had let me know about the incident at school prior to our second session together. He walked reluctantly into the room looking at his feet, his manner markedly different to when I first met him. I let him know that his mother had let me know about an incident at school and that it sounded like it must have been really upsetting for him. I said I imagined that he'd had to talk about this with his parents and teachers and understood that this might have been hard. I explained that I would be curious to hear about his perspective if he wanted to share this with me, while reminding him that he could choose to share as much or as little as he liked. He appeared more relaxed and slowly began to talk about what had happened.

LUCY

Lucy provided some psychoeducation to Gabriel and his family who were attending their second session, explaining that everyone feels angry sometimes and that it was an important emotion. She then proceeded to focus on Gabriel's anger, spending the next half an hour or so eliciting information about the frequency of his anger, how his anger presented, what triggered his anger, and identifying anything that helped when he was angry. Gabriel became increasingly reluctant to participate in this conversation, though his parents were engaged and continued to provide details about his aggressive behavior. Lucy remained focused on collecting information and did not notice that Gabriel was becoming anxious and angry until he stood up and stormed out of the room, bumping the table as he went. In supervision we were able to unpack this and help Lucy understand what she might be able to do differently.

Overtly explaining from the beginning that you are going to help the child as well as their grownups confirms the role of both in the therapy process. It is also often helpful to explain how you will communicate around behaviors. I gently let children know when their grownups have shared information about behaviors in the manner outlined in the example above. It can also be helpful to explain that your role is around more than behavior. For example, I will often tell children that my role is to get to know them so that I can help them to do the things that are important to them and support others to understand them. This is a supportive explanation and, when paired with genuine warmth, respect and curiosity, helps children to understand that your focus will be on so much more than their behavior.

Engaging with the child through play can also help to create safety, as does learning about them more generally. Finding out non-problem-related information helps the child to understand that you value them as a person and builds relationship and safety, helping the child to feel more comfortable in sharing the difficult parts with you. Providing children with choice throughout intervention is also important. Even small choices, such as asking which color marker they would like or whether they would like to draw on the whiteboard or on paper can serve to reinforce their autonomy. The other choice I often explain, as noted above, is that they can tell me as much or as little as they choose.

Setting up expectations around how you can communicate around anger, behaviors and the like is also helpful. Children who struggle to regulate their anger often receive negative attention both at home and at school, and coming to therapy can feel like an extension of this. It may be perceived as another space in which they will be "told off" for doing the wrong thing or a punishment for being "bad." They commonly view their anger as bad and shameful and may be reluctant to talk about it. Part of the therapeutic process, however, does sometimes involve talking about the difficult things, and it is important that you create a space in which both children and their grownups are able to do so. For example, talking with the grownups about when and how they can let you know about angry outbursts helps to orientate them to how you will work together. Your knowledge of the family will guide how you do this.

With grownups who can share concerns about the child in a respectful manner, balancing these with positive reflections and taking responsibility for their own role in any challenges, it might work well to touch base all together at the beginning of a session. On the other hand, for grownups who are struggling to understand and manage their child's anger and describe challenges in a blaming manner, you are likely to need to set up a separate time to communicate about this. When you see the child and their grownups separately, thinking about how you communicate what you learn from one to the other is also important.

These discussions are important to have in the context of talking about confidentiality more generally; however, in practice most children are happy for you to communicate themes from their sessions, and it can be helpful to acknowledge what grownups have shared in the manner outlined above. Suggesting some ways you might manage this as you begin therapy and continuing to check in around this process throughout is recommended.

Creating a space that promotes respectful exploration of a child's anger begins with our first sessions. Most therapists have an introduction they use with children, adapting this to the child's developmental level. For children with emotional regulation difficulties and aggression, I would recommend including the following points in your introduction: that everyone gets angry at times and that anger is an important feeling, that lots of children find anger difficult and that your job is to help children better understand their anger so that they can choose how they respond to it.

Equally important is how we put this into practice. What we say needs to match what we do or we risk, as in the example of Lucy above, rupturing our relationship with the child and family. While ruptures and the process of repair can be valuable in therapy, we tend to be better positioned to navigate this with children and families when we are further into the therapy process. Embodying what we say, both about feelings generally and about anger specifically, allows us to work authentically. If we communicate that all feelings are normal and valuable, yet don't lean in and explore a child's or grownup's uncomfortable feelings, then we are not acting authentically. The same is true if we articulate that everyone gets angry then only proceed to explore the child's anger, rather than giving some examples of our own and exploring the grownups' anger, as in the example of Lucy above. Embodying what we want the child to understand about anger and uncomfortable feelings more generally is powerful and effective.

Assessing a child's emotional awareness and regulation skills

OSCAR

Oscar (8 years) readily entered the clinic room and began playing with the toys. When engaged in play with me he was able to use some feeling words, like sad and happy, and could name what made him feel this way. He found it hard to link these feelings with what he experienced in his body and what might be going through his head. Oscar also found it hard to talk about a broader range of feelings, including anger, which was the primary concern for his grandmother who had brought him to the appointment.

An important part of our assessment involves developing a sense of a child's emotional awareness and regulation skills. Exploration of their anger is best undertaken in the context of exploring their emotions more generally. Some of this information can be gathered by talking to children and grownups, while other parts are best garnered through clinical observation. Having a good understanding of their emotional awareness and regulation skills helps us to structure our intervention appropriately.

Positioning anger as just one of the many emotions to be explored takes away some of the power of this emotion and can reframe the way the child relates to anger, reinforcing the idea that it is an emotion like any other. It also allows you to balance the assessment process, learning about other feelings and developing a more holistic view of the child. Learning about what makes a child happy, for example, often allows us to explore a child's interests and resources, helping us to build a relationship with them and enabling us to identify any tools that might be useful in the therapy process.

Exploring the full range of emotions also allows us to identify the language the child uses around feelings and develop insight into their emotional awareness and regulation abilities.

Noticing how a child talks about emotions is crucial. For example, do they have language around emotions and do they appear comfortable when discussing feelings? Is the language nuanced, with the child using words like "a little" or "a lot" or different descriptors, such as "annoyed" or "furious," to indicate the extent of their feeling? Noticing whether a child finds it challenging to talk about their anger, despite being able to talk about more comfortable feelings, such as happiness, is also telling. Children who come to therapy often lack a language around emotions and appear visibly uncomfortable talking about emotions. They may become engaged with something different to avoid talking about feelings or may even become dysregulated and angry in the session.

Understanding how a child connects their own experience with emotions is also essential. For example, is the child able to say what they notice in their body when they experience an emotion? Can they reflect on when particular feelings come up for them? Are they aware of how they typically respond in these situations or the thoughts that go through their head? Some children will be far more attuned to their experience than others, and many, such as the child in the example above, will require some support during the therapy process to develop these skills.

Children may not be able to articulate their beliefs about emotions; however, these can often be observed in the room. For example, children may have a belief that anger is inappropriate and should be suppressed. A child who believes this might look nervously at their grownup when you ask about anger or might say that they never get angry. Alternatively, they may see anger as justified and something that can be used against others as needed. These children will quickly offer explanations for times that they were angry, attributing this to others. There may be other beliefs that relate to therapy too. For example, children will sometimes have a belief that others need to stop making them angry rather than that they need to find more appropriate ways of expressing their anger. Beliefs such as these are often not overtly expressed; however, it is important for the therapist to maintain a curiosity around these and consider how they can create different experiences. Often these beliefs occur in the context of the family, so understanding how a child's view of self, others and the world has been formed can often help us gain insight into their beliefs around emotion.

As always, your observations of a child in the room are essential. More general observations around how a child plays and relates to you and their family in the space can often help you understand a lot about them. How they approach talking about anger and other feelings is also very telling. For example, a child who suddenly becomes very distracted when you engage them in an activity about emotions is communicating their discomfort with feelings and is providing us with just as much valuable clinical information as if they were to complete the task. Being alert to what is happening in the room is essential and allows us to adapt our approach so that we can gradually help them feel more comfortable with feelings.

Assessing coping and calming

First sessions provide an opportunity to assess the child's coping skills and calming strategies. Children who have angry outbursts often lack coping skills or utilize maladaptive strategies (Braet *et al.* 2014; Carlson *et al.* 2023), and exploring this allows us to identify both resources as well as any needs a child has in this space.

Children will often have some calming strategies that they are using, though these are not always recognized by their families. For example, a child may find gaming or reading calming; however, a grownup may not recognize that aspect, viewing this as simply a leisure activity. This is particularly true when children engage in active calming strategies, such as jumping on a trampoline. Using curiosity to explore what a child finds calming early in therapy is often helpful, both noticing what they find regulating in the room and learning from them and their grownups about what they do at home. Drawing on existing calming strategies more often is an easy and effective intervention.

It is also important to recognize that a child may enlist a range of unhelpful or maladaptive coping responses. They may, for example, turn anger upon a sibling in the form of verbal aggression or may smash and break things when angry. Understanding these patterns helps us to recognize the need and begin to think about how we can build more effective coping skills. For example, the child who turns their distress and anger on a sibling is likely to benefit from being able to express their feelings with the support of a grownup, while a child who tends to break things when angry is likely to need some physical calming strategies.

First sessions with grownups

As with children, it is essential that we spend our first sessions getting to know the grownups, building a relationship with them, learning about their family, and laying the groundwork for therapy. Assessment should involve generally getting to know the family and finding out about the child's early history and current functioning, as well as family functioning more broadly. This section outlines some considerations related specifically to emotional regulation and anger, rather than providing a more general outline of what is needed in an assessment.

Exploring grownups' own experiences of anger

LIAM

Liam had grown up with a father who drank frequently and was prone to violent outbursts. These outbursts were unpredictable and scary for Liam and he grew up learning that anger was unsafe. As a parent, Liam was very patient with his own children and found his wife's anger at their son's aggressive behavior very upsetting. His wife felt unsupported by Liam's very passive responses to their son and would become even more angry in this context, often shouting or slamming a door and further triggering Liam. When engaged in parenting work the therapist was able to support Liam and his wife to understand their own experiences of anger and commit to finding safe ways of expressing anger within their family.

EZRA

Ezra was a single parent whose daughter was autistic and had significant emotional regulation difficulties. Upon commencing therapy, the therapist encouraged her to talk about her own feelings about her daughter's anger and to consider her own early experiences of anger. Ezra often made significant comments around this toward the end of the first few sessions, such as reflecting on how critical her own mother had been and touching on her own anger and grief around her daughter's challenges. She would then move the conversation away from these areas, focusing again on her concerns for her daughter. Acknowledging these important comments and gently returning to these in subsequent sessions enabled Ezra to explore these experiences and how they shaped her current responses to her daughter at a pace that felt safe for her.

A grownup's own regulation influences both the way they will model managing feelings for their child and how supportive they can be in response to the child's emotions (Hajal and Paley 2020). Implicit in this is the idea that children's experiences are likely to vary and are important to explore as we get to know a child and family. Grownups have their own experiences of anger and often have well-established beliefs around the emotion and ways of responding when it arises. Understanding this is obviously helpful in our work with children and families; however, grownups can find this challenging, particularly early in the therapy process. As therapists, we are faced with a difficult balance of knowing enough to begin working with the child and family and appreciating that grownups often need to let this story unfold over time.

Grownups who bring their child to therapy can find it anxiety-provoking to have the focus shift to themselves and their own experiences, which means that child therapists need to approach this thoughtfully. Orientating the family to this right from the beginning is helpful. It is often helpful to provide some examples of how grownups' own experiences of anger can shape the way in which they respond to their children as a way of opening up this conversation and providing a rationale for exploring this space.

It is also important to pace this for the family, finding a balance between keeping this a focus and allowing the family to explore this as they feel able to do so. As in the example of Ezra above, we often need to allow grownups to share this story over time, gradually deepening their awareness as therapy progresses. For us as therapists, this sometimes means that we need to sit with the uncertainty of not having a complete understanding of the situation and trust that this will become clearer over time.

We also need to recognize that talking about their own feelings and thoughts can be incredibly confronting for grownups. They may, for example, feel uncomfortable acknowledging some of the thoughts and feelings that come up when they are angry or feel terrified by the similarities between their own behavior and that of their child or their own grownups. It can be easy as a therapist to get caught up in a grownup's avoidance. We might, for example, follow a grownup's lead and stay focused on their child's behavior, missing an important piece of the picture. Maintaining an awareness of this and gently circling back from time to time, expressing a curiosity about how this might be having an impact on how they are able to support their child can be helpful. Sometimes, in therapy, we do find ourselves becoming stuck and needing to pause and reassess so that we can better understand what is happening for the child and family. If you need to further explore a grownup's early experiences it is often easier to pivot and return to this if you have touched on this during your first sessions.

Helping the family to understand their experiences around anger and articulate their beliefs about the emotion, supporting them to consider whether or not this is working for them as a family, is an important part of therapy. If a family's experience is that anger is internalized rather than expressed, they can be encouraged to explore how this is working for their child. With openness and curiosity, we can consider together whether this works for their child, supporting them to consider both the short-term and long-term implications of this. We can wonder with the family about how this aligns with their values and what they want for their child, identifying any aspects that they may want to reconsider.

Feelings about feelings are very relevant in our work with families. In a narrower sense we might consider the feelings that come up around a particular emotion, such as anger, as discussed above. In a broader sense, however, Gottman *et al.* (1996) point out that the construct allows us to understand how families might engage with emotions more generally, noting that some will welcome a broad range of feelings, while others may see these as something to be avoided and minimized. Having an awareness of how the family engages with emotions more generally is helpful to explore in the first sessions with the child and family.

We have reflected on how a family's experiences shape the way in which they express and respond to expressions of anger, and it is important to acknowledge that cultural background and religion may be a part of this. Exploring this openly rather than making generalizations based on a child and family's cultural group or religious identification is essential.

Understanding grownups' responses and reflective capacity

PRIYA

After the third session with Priya and her grandmother, I received an email in which her grandmother shared some moments of connection they had shared over the school break. Until then, I had only heard about Priya's challenges and the difficult moments and had been trying to thicken the narrative and explore some of the good times. I smiled broadly as I read the more balanced story in this email. My smile was not diminished as I read the next email, which came through a couple of days later, and again focused on Priya's angry outbursts. What I had glimpsed was a small shift and, even though it had yet to be maintained, its presence reassured me that we were moving toward seeing Priya's strengths as well as her challenges.

FLORA

Flora tentatively acknowledged that her voice might get louder when her son was dysregulated, looking at me cautiously. She seemed relieved when reassured that I would be surprised if she was completely calm when her son was so angry, and we were able to explore what her own feelings might tell her about what her son was experiencing. In the following session Flora shared that she sometimes became furious in response to her anger and was able to talk about the shame she experienced around this as well as her worry about sharing this.

Assessing how the grownups view their child's angry behavior is an important aspect to explore during the assessment stage, and exploring how this relates to a parent's other experiences of anger is also often important. It's crucial to understand how the grownups make sense of the child's anger and what thoughts or worries come up for them when their child is angry. These ideas may be clearly formed, such as "He's just like me when I was younger," or they may be more tentative, for example "Sometimes I think this has something to do with her being bullied last year at school." When we have a belief, our natural tendency is to look for information that confirms this. If a grownup's belief is that that child is always angry and oppositional then they may miss information to the contrary. Missing those moments when their child manages challenges well or expresses anger appropriately further exacerbates the challenges for the family, often leaving them very stuck. Recognizing the lens through which children are seen is therefore important.

During first sessions, it's helpful to have children and grownups share their narrative about the problem. Rather than simply adopting the narrative, as therapists we weave these understandings together and may introduce other possible interpretations, enriching and creating a deeper understanding. Sometimes the narrative can be very far removed from the present moment. For example, a parent once surprised me by explaining that when her 10-year-old had angry outbursts she worried that he was going to become a drug addict and a criminal. Uncovering this thought and worry helped me to better understand the magnitude and tenor of her response in a way I don't think would have been possible without this knowledge. It opened up further exploration about her experiences of anger and her beliefs about this emotion.

Understanding how the grownups currently respond to their child's emotions and what they are doing that helps or doesn't help is also useful. Slowing these discussions down so that you can really understand what happens between the grownup and the child is important, and it is essential that the discussion focuses on the grownup too. This can be challenging, however. Parents who bring their child for therapy implicitly identify the problem as being with the child and may be unprepared to reflect upon their own role. As therapists, we need to manage this carefully. Helping the family understand from the beginning that they will all play an active role in therapy should help; however, having lots of empathy along the way will also create safety for grownups and allow them to share more openly with you. I will often make statements like "That must be so hard to have her responding like that" or "It sounds incredibly difficult." Comments like this acknowledge the grownup's experience and create a space for grownups to talk openly about how they respond in the moment, even when this is different to how they know they should respond or how they would like to respond.

Understanding the feelings that arise for a grownup when their child is angry is important. It gives us some insight into anything we might need to explore further with the family. Helpfully though, it also gives us some insight into a grownup's own regulation. For example, do they feel angry and respond quickly by yelling? Or are they able to feel the anger and take some breaths to settle themselves, allowing them to empathize with their child? Understanding these responses is crucial as we want to move toward grownups being able to regulate themselves so they can support their children to do so.

Grownups will often identify strategies they use when they describe how they respond to their child's anger. It can be tempting to accept a strategy they talk about using at face value, noting it down and moving into fixing mode by attempting to think of an alternative approach. It is essential, however, that we really slow this conversation down so that we can understand moment to moment what happens in their interaction with the child. This helps us really understand what is happening and enables us to look at this from a regulation point of view. We might say something like "So it sounds like you take some big breaths and try to calm yourself before suggesting that he go to his room. What happens then?" You can also normalize how challenging the situation might be and provide a space for the grownups to talk about inconsistencies. For example, you might say something along the lines of "Most people find there are times when they struggle to stay calm and don't use the strategies they normally would, such as sending their child to their room. I wonder if you ever have that experience."

It is also very helpful to assess a grownup's capacity to reflect on what is happening for their child in the moment. Asking what a grownup thinks might be happening for their child when they are angry can be useful. Questions like "What do you think was going on for her?" are useful in eliciting the grownup's thoughts about this; however, they also give us some insight about the grownup's capacity for mentalization. A grownup who responds that they have "no idea" is likely to need a different approach in therapy to a grownup who can share some wonderings based on their knowledge of the child and has spent some time reflecting on this. We can also ask about what they think their child most needs when they are angry.

When a grownup finds it hard to mentalize about their child, it is often helpful to try to understand why this is difficult. For example, it might be that the grownup has a good sense of the child and has previously been able to consider their perspective, though is experiencing particularly high levels of stress at present or is struggling with their own mental health. It might be that the grownup was attuned to a child previously, though began to struggle as a child entered a new developmental stage. At other times it becomes apparent that the grownup has always struggled to consider the perspective of their child or that they find it very challenging when their child's feelings are different to their own. Sometimes this might relate to a grownup's own attachment history or even a neurodiverse thinking pattern.

The box below includes some questions that are often useful to explore with grownups. These questions and observations provide insight into a grownup's ability to think about their child's needs and gives you insight into their ability to co-regulate the child. For some families, these questions precipitate some new understandings and will, in and of themselves, form the beginning of therapeutic change.

Helpful questions for grownups

What leads to an angry outburst?

What does an angry outburst usually look like?

When your child is angry, what do they do/look like/say?

When they are angry, what is this like for you? What do you do/look like/say?

What are the thoughts/worries that come up for you when your child is angry?

What are the feelings/memories that come up for you when your child is angry?

How long does an outburst usually last?

How do others respond to the angry outburst?

What happens just prior to the outburst ceasing?

What does your child most need when they are angry?

Is there anything your child finds calming when they are angry?

How do you make sense of the anger?

What do you think is going on for your child?

What happens when you get angry? What about others in your family?

What would you like your child to know about anger?

How would you like anger to be managed in your family?

General family functioning

More generally, it can be useful to have an understanding of how the family functions. Having a broader sense of a grownup's mental health often helps. It's also helpful to know what the family enjoys, how they spend time together and what their days and weeks look like. It is also useful to know about any pressures and stresses as well as about any traumatic or formative experiences they may have had in the past. Understanding a grownup's support network, having a sense of their resources, as well as how they manage self-care, can also be helpful.

It is important to understand a grownup's overall level of stress and whether they experience their own emotional regulation difficulties or mental health challenges. Clinically, grownups who struggle to regulate their own emotions often experience difficulty responding to uncomfortable expressions of emotion in their children. Research is beginning to explore these relationships and generally supports the need to consider how a grownup's own emotion regulation impacts on their ability to respond sensitively to their child's uncomfortable emotions (Bertie, Johnston and Lill 2021; Carreras *et al.* 2019). Therefore, while it is not the role of child therapists to treat a grownup's mental health issues, we may need to identify these concerns, helping the grownup to understand how these might relate to their parenting and supporting them to access their own therapy.

Understanding how the family functions helps us to best support them. Knowing whether there are frequent conflicts over behavior management, for example, might mean that you work to ensure that all of the child's grownups are involved in the process of therapy. It can also be helpful to understand what sort of rhythms or routines the family tends to have across their days. Sometimes it becomes clear that the child is over-scheduled and that building calming rhythms will support regulation. In Chapter 4 we talk more about supporting grownups to include calming rhythms across the child's day.

Openness to different ideas

Being actively involved in therapy can be challenging for many grownups. Most are juggling multiple demands and many have their own difficulties. In first sessions it can often be helpful to get a sense of a grownup's ability to engage with their child in a different way or try something new. For me, this usually starts with a wondering.

I might wonder, for example, what would happen if we could catch a child as he began to become dysregulated or if we could offer some calming options to a child prior to engaging with her in talking about behavior. Some grownups will respond to these wonderings with curiosity; they may have questions about what I mean or how that could be helpful. They may even go away and try this with the child between sessions. Others will respond by telling me they have tried that or that it doesn't work. Posing these ideas as a curiosity in the context of already having built a bit of a relationship with the grownup usually allows them to tell me what they think. If I feel they are holding back, however, I might ask about their thoughts or notice that they are looking skeptical and express my interest in learning why. Sometimes, in sharing their reservations, grownups will share more about what works for their child and will come away with a different approach they are curious to try with their child. This is a wonderful outcome and provides an opportunity for me to notice how much they know about their child and how important they are in this process. For others, however, this process can help us uncover some of the challenges to engaging in therapy, such as a sense of hopelessness around the child's anger or parental exhaustion.

Having a better sense of this can help us to pace therapy for the family, meeting them where they are at. It ensures that we don't risk the therapeutic relationship by not creating a shared understanding first or by asking them to do things they are not ready to do or are yet not capable of doing.

Keeping first sessions play-based

ALEX

Alex came in for his first session with his father. His father began the session by encouraging Alex to talk about his angry outbursts. Alex responded by staring at his feet, twisting the toe of his shoe into the floor. I wondered aloud whether this might be hard to talk about and suggested we do something else first to help Alex settle into the session. Later in the session, I introduced a feelings game, suggesting that we all take turns and share about our feelings on our turn. Alex engaged well in this game and I was able to learn about his experience of anger in addition to understanding the shame he felt around this.

It is important that when assessing we don't slip into just talking, as doing so might limit the child's ability to share their experience and demonstrate their emotional awareness. Rather, we need to provide developmentally appropriate ways in which a child can share their world with us. The assessment activities included here provide some playful ways of better understanding a child's experience of anger. You can use these activities with or without grownups present, depending on your clinical judgment and the structure of the assessment. Where grownups are present, it is often helpful to involve them in the activity. My preferred way of doing this is to have them complete their own version of the activity, which is often incredibly normalizing for the child. This is also a good opportunity to talk with the grownup about what emotional examples might be shared during sessions and will give you a good sense of whether the child and their grownups can work together in this way or whether some other work is needed first.

You will notice that some of these activities encourage a broader conversation around emotions, rather than simply on anger. As discussed, this allows us to understand a child's emotional awareness more generally and communicates the idea that all feelings are important and valuable, including anger. My co-authored book *Creative Ways to Help Children Manage Big Feelings* (Zandt and Barrett 2017) includes a number of other activities that can be used in this way and can be particularly useful for children who find it hard to talk about emotions.

Some of the activities aim to assess and begin building a child's awareness of their anger, increasing their noticing skills. I use the concept of inside and outside noticing to explain this to children, explaining that inside noticing involves being aware of anything that is happening inside of you and includes any feelings, bodily sensations and thoughts. It may also include ideas, daydreams or urges; anything that is an internal experience and cannot be seen by another person is relevant here. I then explain that outside noticing involves tuning into your environment. This can include noticing sights, sounds and smells in your physical world. It can also include noticing another person. You might, for example, notice how another person's face is looking or how their body is moving.

Some of the activities explore a child's coping skills or regulation skills. These activities may uncover unrecognized resources or help identify unhelpful coping skills, which grownups may have presumed to be misbehavior. The activities also provide a space to explore how the child's grownups regulate, helping them develop more awareness of this and supporting you to identify strengths as well as areas that might need to be a focus. These activities are useful as you move into therapy, ensuring that the family has some skills they can draw on as needed.

Many of these activities are therapeutic in and of themselves, reminding us again that assessments and therapy sit along a continuum. Sometimes, in first sessions, you can feel the desire to jump into intervention and offer strategies or provide psychoeducation. While it can be helpful to have some gentle wonderings or observations that deepen the family's understanding of the challenges in the first sessions, moving too quickly into the intervention space is often unhelpful. When we offer strategies too early we risk doing this in a way that doesn't fit for the family, and we increase the likelihood that these ideas will be rejected or implemented in an unhelpful way, causing us to need to repair the relationship or leading to the family disengaging. Noticing your own thoughts and feelings during first sessions is crucial, and supervision is a useful space for exploring this. It is often preferable to observe which ideas a child picks up on from these activities and notice how they integrate this. These observations can tell us a lot about how the child is likely to engage in therapy and can help us to plan more effectively as we move into therapy.

My anger is...

This activity is a useful one in the assessment phase, allowing children to explore their anger, putting words, colors and shapes to it.

What you need
A selection of magazines, newspapers, different colored and textured papers, markers or pencils, scissors and glue.

Introducing this activity
You can introduce this activity by suggesting that you all make a collage about what anger is like for each of you and showing them the materials and explaining that they can cut and paste to create a picture about their anger. If a child seems unsure, you might provide a reflection about how this can feel difficult or not knowing where to start, depending on what seems appropriate. You may like to begin demonstrating with your own collage, showing the child, for example, that you are choosing a toaster because you often feel hot when you are angry. You can also show the child that you can draw or write words using markers in addition to or instead of cutting and pasting.

It is often useful to see what the child identifies with spontaneously in this activity, and the amount of detail in the collage often speaks to how well a child understands their anger. If it is appropriate, however, to prompt the child, you might like to use some of the following prompts to support the child in their search for items to draw or paste. These could include what color the child's anger is like, if there are any animals the child's anger reminds them of, if there is a particular type of weather that fits with their angry feeling. Having grownups create their own collage is often valuable too, providing a useful model for the child and helping you to have a better understanding of their experience too. Notice what the child includes in their collage and what this tells you about how they experience anger in their body, what they tend to do when they are angry, and what their thoughts about anger are.

When the collage has been created you can ask a child to share what they notice. They may also like to share what they notice when looking at your picture or their grownup's picture.

Considerations and adaptations
If you are working online, collages can readily be created in a document by copying and pasting in images found on the internet. Children may need greater levels of scaffolding when working online as they won't have pictures in front of them, so the above prompts can be helpful.

Children are often happy to take their picture home, which can help them to continue the discussion within their families.

What's bugging you?

This activity was inspired by Paris Goodyear-Brown's *Worry worm* activity (2010) and Karen Treisman's (2017, 2020) *Things that bug me…* worksheet. In a similar way I draw on the metaphor about being bugged to help the child articulate what is annoying them.

What you need
Small plastic bug toys, the kind that are readily available in toy stores or online, and a sandtray.

Introducing this activity
To introduce this I show the child the bugs and ask about whether they have ever heard the saying "It's bugging me." We talk together about what that means as we look at the bugs and I suggest that we hide the bugs in some sand and name something that bugs us as we find them. Younger and older children generally understand this metaphor, though you may need to be more overt about it with children who tend to be quite literal.

A sandtray is helpful for this, and I find that the sand is quite regulating for lots of children, which helps them to share more of what is bothering them. If you don't have a sandtray you could hide the bugs in some Play-Doh, a tray of rice or something similar. Obviously, if you have a child who finds textures like this challenging, you might like to simply hide the bugs around the room.

Asking the child's grownups about what bugs them as you introduce this activity is often helpful and is a good way to include them in this. I find that children really enjoy this activity and are often quite happy to look for the bugs on their own and name something that annoys them. If they are reluctant to do so, however, you can always take turns to find the bugs and name something. I also encourage grownups to take a turn and name something that bugs them. If you are working online you could send some bug pictures to the family ahead of time and ask the grownup to cut these up so they could be hidden.

Considerations and adaptations
This game often has a good flow and children enjoy finding the bugs as quickly as they can. Stopping and talking about each annoying thing they name might not be clinically appropriate in this context; however, you can note this and return to it when they have found all of the bugs. Children might like to draw some bugs afterwards while you reflect on this further. Encouraging them to draw the biggest bug and name the biggest thing that bugs them can also be helpful. If you are working online, you might like to have the child draw pictures of bugs on an online whiteboard or look at some pictures of bugs while you chat about this together.

Engaging grownups in conversation about whether they knew these things bugged the child, what it is they notice when the child is annoyed and how they can help support the child when these things happen is often helpful.

Children may like to take their picture with them or even take a plastic bug with them if you have extras on hand. This can sometimes prompt further noticing of small triggers at home and help grownups to be more attuned to their child's overall level of regulation.

The shape of my anger

This activity is useful for encouraging children to reflect more on their anger and understand the form it typically takes.

What you need

Paper and markers or pencils.

Introducing this activity

To introduce this I usually suggest to the child that we might draw anger while we talk about it. I generally complete this one alongside children, given that it is more abstract in nature, so explaining that I will draw my anger too I begin to reflect on what color I might use and encourage the child to do likewise. I may engage with the child in some discussion about the color they chose and why it is a good fit for their anger; however, for children who are ready to draw or are focused on the task at hand I am likely to leave these questions till later.

Having chosen a color I begin wondering about what sort of shape the child's anger might be. Empathizing with this feeling and encouraging them to try drawing and see what comes up is often helpful. If the child is still unsure, I might suggest some examples, giving them a few options to encourage their own ideas. For example, I might say "Well, sometimes anger might be hard to hold like a great messy squiggly shape." For other people, it comes up quickly, and it might be a strong shape that fills the whole page. Others might find that their anger rises suddenly though it takes a long time to pass so they might make a shape with a very long tail. I will often draw the shape of my anger and encourage grownups to draw one for themselves too, which can also provide a helpful model for the child. Younger children may need more support with this activity and may need to draw the shape in collaboration with their grownup, who can share their observations to support this reflection.

When the shapes have been drawn, we reflect together on what we notice about these. Ensuring that the reflection fits with the child's language skills is important. I generally find that it is helpful to add one or two things to the child's reflection, keeping in mind that adding more may be too challenging for the child. In these situations you may like to share further reflections with the grownup. Reflections might include what happens in a child's body when they are angry, what happens and how they tend to interact with others when they are angry, what tends to lead to this anger, and what helps.

Considerations and adaptations

Older children are likely to be able to reflect more on their experience of anger. For example, it may be helpful to encourage them to notice what thought patterns they experience in this context.

When reflecting with grownups, you might like to talk about how their anger shape relates to the child's. Positioning the pictures together is a visual way to demonstrate this interaction. Encouraging children to take the pictures home and talk to another grownup or even an older sibling about these is likely to be helpful.

This activity can readily be completed online using an online whiteboard or having the child draw at home and show you their picture. You can also use pipe-cleaners for this activity for children who might prefer this option, having the child bend these to illustrate the shape of their anger.

Rainbow pom-pom feelings

This simple activity encourages children to talk about their feelings, including their angry feelings. It helps children to see their angry feelings as just one of their many feelings and supports them to express these. Making pom-poms is generally relaxing and pairing this with talking about feelings often supports children to share more about their experience of emotions.

What you need
Cardboard, scissors and different colors of wool.

Introducing this activity
To create a pom-pom you will need two circles of cardboard, each with a smaller circle cut out inside of it as in Figure 2.1. You could trace some circular items or use a compass to create your cardboard template, which should look like a donut. Sandwich the two pieces of cardboard together and show the child how you can wrap the wool around, as in Figure 2.1.

As you add each color, encourage the child to think of a feeling that color reminds them of. Allow the child to wrap the wool around as they tell you about that feeling. For example, you can encourage the child to talk about what they notice in their body when they have that feeling and about a time they felt that way. Older children might also like to share what their thoughts were as they recall a time when they felt angry. Complete this process again for other feelings, using a different color of wool for each. It is helpful to be guided by the emotions the child identifies here; however, if they are unable to list a mix of both comfortable and uncomfortable feelings, you might like to prompt some of these. Try to have a mix of happy, sad, angry and worried feelings, using whatever words the child uses for these feelings. When the child can no longer identify any further feelings, you can return to those feelings you have already covered, adding another piece of wool as you talk about these again. Ideally, you want to wrap the donut shape two or three times with the wool.

When this has been done, take the scissors, as pictured in Figure 2.1, and gently insert these between the two cardboard pieces on the outer edge of the donut shape, carefully cutting the wool along the outer edge whilst still holding carefully to ensure the pom-pom stays together. Holding the middle of the pom-pom together, tie another piece of wool between the two cardboard pieces as in Figure 2.1 and pull it tight before tying a knot in it. Ease the pieces of cardboard off as in Figure 2.1 and gently fluff out the pom-pom. Most grownups don't have the materials for this activity on hand, so if I were using this activity online, I would make this as I am engaging with a child, having them choose the colors and telling me how much. I would then put it aside to give to them the next time they come in or mail it to them following the session.

As you look together at the pom-pom, you might like to notice all of the colors with the child and comment on how they all look together, emphasizing the idea that all of our feelings are part of the overall creation. You might like to encourage the child and grownup to keep the pom-pom somewhere handy and check in around any feelings they notice when they see it.

Considerations and adaptations

Grownups can be encouraged to support the child as they talk about these emotions. Alternatively, you might like to have grownups make their own pom-pom alongside the child, adding the same colors the child does though reflecting on their own feelings.

It can be helpful to have your cardboard ready ahead of time, particularly with younger children. It is also important to keep in mind that younger children or those with fine motor difficulties might find the fine motor aspects of this task challenging and may need support with this.

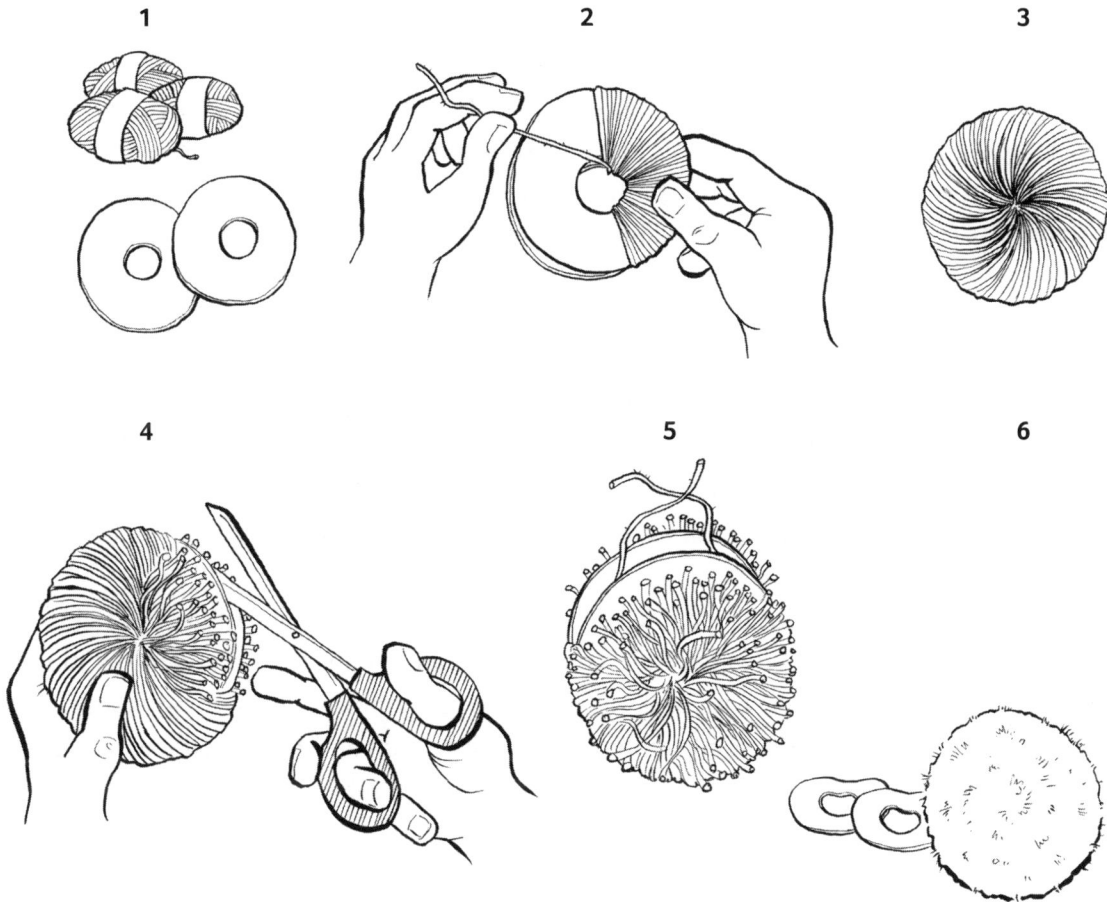

FIGURE 2.1 HOW TO MAKE A POM-POM

Angry puppet stories

This is a useful activity for understanding how a child responds to and feels about anger in a developmentally appropriate way.

What you need
Some hand or finger puppets.

Introducing this activity
To begin this activity, I show the child the puppets and allow them to lead the play to begin with. Sometimes children will bring emotions into the play spontaneously; however, if they don't, I might introduce some emotional content through the puppets. For example, I might say something like "This is Danny the Dog. He loves bones and digging holes. Danny doesn't like the cat next door." I will then pause and notice how the child responds. I will often then introduce some emotions into the play, often beginning with comfortable feelings. For example, I might enact Danny's feelings when he gets a bone. I'll notice if the child names these feelings and how they respond, before introducing uncomfortable feelings, including anger. Doing this through the puppets, such as having the dog bark angrily in response to seeing a cat close by, allows children to explore these angry feelings and allows us to develop a sense of their emotional awareness. Noticing how grownups respond to these scenarios is also helpful. Looking out for any emotional regulation strategies that a child includes in the play is also valuable.

Some children will spontaneously become very engaged in the play while others will be hesitant to do so, preferring to observe. Whispering to the child about what is happening in the play and asking for their input this way can be helpful. You might, for example, say something more general, like "Oh no… what now?" or even something more specific, such as "What is Danny going to do now?" to invite greater involvement whilst still allowing a child to feel comfortable.

Considerations and adaptations
If the child enjoys the activity and is engaged with this, you might encourage them to tell a story with another puppet that includes some angry feelings. Grownups can also be asked to tell a story that includes some angry feelings, which can also provide insight into how they understand and manage this emotion. Alternatively, you can use another puppet to tell a different story, again including both comfortable and uncomfortable feelings.

Younger children seem particularly interested in puppet play, though older children will sometimes enjoy this too. The language you use when playing can readily be modified to ensure that it is appropriate to the child you are working with. If you are working online, you can still encourage the child to direct the story as you enact it in front of the camera. You can also encourage children to use their stuffed toys to create a story for you.

When reflecting on this activity it can be helpful to notice how children responded to emotions and explore how this relates to their challenges with anger. Sharing observations of the grownups may also be relevant in this context.

Bang it out

This activity helps children to name and begin scaling their anger.

What you need
The boardgame Don't Break the Ice.

Introducing this activity
When playing Don't Break the Ice in the traditional way, players tap cubes of ice with small hammers. The aim of the game is to knock as few cubes out at a time as possible, which becomes increasingly hard as the game progresses. Whoever topples the penguin standing in the middle of the ice loses.

You can play a game or two in the above manner, before suggesting that the child could name something that makes them angry as they tap. I suggest that the child tap to show how angry they feel, with a small tap for things that make them a little angry and bigger, harder, tapping for those things that make them more angry. This allows the child to engage through their body and helps us notice body changes. I will often comment on this as we are playing, noticing, for example, "Wow that was a big one! You knocked down five blocks. I could see the anger on your face looking really mad and your words got faster and louder." Naming these experiences not only helps the child to connect with what is happening in their body, it also supports family members to tune in to their child's experience, helping them to notice when the child is becoming angry and encourages empathy.

Grownups can readily be involved in this game, taking turns with the child, and sharing examples of their own anger as they take a turn. They can also provide scaffolding should the child need help to think of an example, tentatively offering suggestions about times when the child has been angry. Younger children may require more support to reflect on this. I will also take turns with the child in playing this game, using incidental teaching to provide examples that support the child's emotional expression. For example, if I notice that the child is not able to name the things that make them angry, I will share some examples that are appropriate to the child's developmental level and notice whether the child connects with any of these examples. For children who readily provide examples of triggers, I might suggest the next time we play that we name something that happens inside of us when we are angry and see how the child responds to this.

Considerations and adaptations
The game Don't Break the Ice is not an exact one. As the game progresses and the ice becomes unstable, children can knock down lots of ice even with a small tap. This may be frustrating for some children, particularly if they have a preference for things being precise. This is, however, a great opportunity to work through any annoyances or frustration, regulating the child as needed.

This activity provides lots of useful information about a child's emotional awareness and regulation skills. You can reflect about what you noticed with the child and grownup, getting curious about how this relates to their anger at home and in other environments.

Inside and outside elastics jump

This activity helps you to assess a child's ability to notice their own experience and those of others. It provides an opportunity to increase their awareness and is particularly helpful for children who are not tuning in to signs that they are becoming angry.

What you need

A set of elastics or a hula hoop. (Elastics are essentially a large loop of elastic and can be purchased quite cheaply, or you can create your own very simply by knotting a long piece of elastic together.) If you don't have another grownup in the session, a hula hoop is a better option as described in the adaptations below.

Introducing this activity

Elastics is an old-fashioned game in which two people stand one to two meters apart positioning a loop of elastic on the outside of their legs. They stand with their legs around half a meter apart, creating a rectangle of elastic between them. A third person then jumps the elastic.

I usually introduce this activity by asking if the child has ever played elastics and if they'd like to try the game. Start with one of the rhymes that children use when they play elastics, such as "England, Ireland, Scotland, Wales, Inside, Outside, Inside, Out"—jumping your feet inside and outside of the elastics with each alternating word. (If you are unfamiliar with playing elastics you might like to look for some examples online.)

Once you have done this you can then start to talk about how the inside and outside jumping reminds you of inside and outside noticing, and then wonder if you can notice something inside when you jump your feet inside the elastics and notice something outside of you when you jump outside of the elastics. If the idea of inside and outside noticing is new for a child and family, you will need to explain further as described earlier in this chapter.

The activation that inevitably comes from jumping over the elastics creates changes in the body, which can readily be noticed and reflected on. For example, the child can be encouraged to notice their breathing, heart rate, or the feeling in their legs as they jump. This is particularly valuable for children who find it difficult to tune in to their bodies and might otherwise struggle to notice what is happening inside of them.

Take turns as you continue the game, each having a go at jumping and offering any other family members who are present a turn. Turn-taking provides an important model, normalizing the child's experience by enabling them to see that the therapist can also have similar experiences. Grownups can be encouraged to participate in the game too.

Considerations and adaptations

If you don't have another grownup in the sessions, a hula hoop can be used for this activity. Create a game of jumping in and out of the hoop, engaging in inside and outside noticing as you do so.

For children who focus solely on one element of their experience, such as their thoughts or the somatic symptoms, your focus with this activity might be around helping them to tune in to other elements of their experience. I might, for example, model noticing thoughts for a child who tends to be very focused on their bodily sensations or describe something I notice about my own body for a child who tends to get caught up in their thoughts. Encouraging the child to do similarly when they have an inside noticing turn often works well. A child's responses will help you to have a sense of their noticing skills, and you can ask about what they notice inside when they are angry. What you model should also remain developmentally appropriate. For example, modeling thoughts works well for older children though not younger children.

When reflecting with the child and family, your focus should be guided by their needs. You might, for example, notice that inside noticing was more difficult and wonder together about how the family might be able to do some of this at home, particularly when the child begins to get upset or angry. Alternatively, you might notice that outside noticing was helpful and wonder how this could be used at times when the child tends to become upset or angry.

Inside and outside noticing dice

This activity also helps you to understand how a child reflects upon their own experiences and those of others, noticing any areas they require further support with. It supports children to increase their awareness and better identify their feelings. It also encourages them to notice what is happening outside of them, providing an opportunity to develop grounding skills and to build on social awareness.

What you need

A foam dice, some paper, scissors and glue or some inexpensive dice and cardboard. You will also need some markers or pencils.

Introducing this activity

You can introduce the idea by suggesting to the child that you make a game together to learn more about them and their feelings. Create a dice which has different inside and outside noticing prompts on each side by writing a selection of the prompts below (see box) on some paper, cutting them out, and sticking one to each side of the dice. You will notice that the prompts vary, allowing you to choose what might work best for the child. Alternatively, give the child a regular dice and create a play card, listing one of the prompts below next to each of the numbers 1–6 so that you can refer to the card as you roll the dice.

When you have created the dice you can take it in turns to roll it, sharing examples on your own turn. Actively involving grownups in this activity is also recommended. Grownups can be encouraged to share their experiences and can support their child to reflect on their experiences.

If a child is finding this activity hard, it is important to scaffold as needed. For example, having a child jump up and down or run around the clinic should help them to notice something in their body. Similarly, being encouraged to look out of a window or taking a walk outside of the clinic can help a child to notice what is happening around them (outside noticing).

It can be helpful as you reflect at the end of the session to think about what the child most needs. Some children need to focus on noticing how they feel, whereas others are overly focused on this, getting caught up in their thoughts and becoming anxious about typical bodily sensations. Having a good sense of the child and their grownups allows you to encourage either inside noticing, outside noticing or some of both, depending on what they most need. You can then encourage the child to focus more on this after they leave the session, helping them to think about how they could do so. Encouraging the child to take the dice home and play with others can help with this too.

Considerations and adaptations

For older children you can choose prompts such as notice one inside thing, notice two outside things, and notice three inside things; however, younger children are likely to need prompts that direct them to specific aspects they can notice, such as one thing they can hear or one thing inside their heart, which often prompts discussion around how they feel or something they desire. Younger children are likely to need you to incorporate greater movement into the activity, so doing something physical between rolls can be helpful and often makes it easier for the child to engage in inside noticing. As always, adapt the wording to choose language that works for the child and family.

If you are working online, you may like to use an online dice and create your play list on an online whiteboard.

Suggested prompts for inside and outside noticing dice

Notice (insert #) inside things.

Notice (insert #) outside things.

Notice one thing inside your body.

Notice one thing inside your head.

Notice one thing in your heart.

Notice one thing you can hear.

Notice one thing you can see.

Notice one thing you can feel.

Notice one thing you can smell.

Notice one thing you can taste.

CHAPTER 3

MOVING INTO THERAPY

In this chapter we talk about the process of moving from assessment into therapy, through creating a shared understanding and developing a therapy plan that meets the needs of the child and family. In addition we focus on how you can monitor the progress of therapy in an ongoing way.

Making sense of it all and coming up with a plan

MARCO

Giulia nodded as I talked with her about how her son Marco's ADHD contributed to his anger. I empathized with how difficult his behavior could be and how Marco's grandmother's tendency to attribute this to "typical boy" behavior had felt invalidating. We talked about how this had led Giulia to increasingly point out Marco's challenges, and I shared my concerns about what this had meant for their relationship. Giulia became tearful and talked about wanting a better relationship with Marco, wondering if sometimes she responded the way she did because he was a bit like his father. I shared that I had wondered this too, given the relationship Giulia had described with Marco's father, who had moved overseas two years previously. Giulia agreed that it had been challenging for Marco to grow up with a father who often shouted and insisted on things being a particular way, and we talked about how this might have shaped the way in which Marco managed his own feelings. We acknowledged that Giulia's focus when the family had lived together was on avoiding upsetting her husband, and we reflected on what this had meant for Marco.

Together, we agreed to work initially on helping Giulia to better understand Marco's ADHD, to create some calming rhythms during the day and to focus on having moments of connection, and we scheduled some parent sessions around this. Giulia decided it would be helpful to talk to her own therapist further about her feelings about Marco's father and explore how this might relate to her parenting as we commenced this work. We also agreed to help Marco develop some further coping skills and begin to notice early signs that he was becoming dysregulated. Giulia agreed to be part of these sessions, which we hoped would help her to regulate Marco more effectively at home, and we talked about using lots of play and movement to keep Marco engaged.

One of the most important skills a therapist can develop is the ability to assess and formulate. A good formulation helps us understand how the problem arose; however, it also helps us identify what the child's and the family's strengths and needs are and how we can best support them with this. It is a nuanced understanding of the family and lays the groundwork for an individualized plan which we can continue revising over time, knowing that assessment and formulation are ongoing. While assessment and therapy are overlapping processes, it is often helpful to mark the movement from your beginning session, in which you are primarily getting to know the child and family, to those sessions in which you focus together on facilitating change. Collaboratively developing an understanding and checking this with the family, as in the example outlined above is helpful.

In addition to knowing what we are going to work on, a good formulation provides us with a sense of how we can work best with the child and family. What follows are some considerations when treatment planning, taking into account the needs of the child and of their grownups.

Working in a way that fits for the child and family
Understanding what the child needs
Bottom-up or top-down?

HEIDI
Heidi (8 years) had completed a block of therapy with each of her parents, which was aimed at helping them engage in a more playful and attuned way. Her parents became more attuned to her and reported more positive interactions at home. In sessions the therapist supported them to co-regulate Heidi, using breathing and sensory strategies as they named and supported her through her feelings. Heidi was naming her feelings in sessions and had started taking a deep breath when she was becoming dysregulated in the clinic room. She was increasingly able to be co-regulated at home; however, she continued to struggle with regulation in times of high anxiety, particularly at school where she would become oppositional and avoidant. Heidi's parents and I agreed that it would be a good time to introduce some cognitive strategies. I noted that Heidi was now more able to put language to her experience, meaning that she could better engage with some of these strategies.

LEVI
Levi came into a session very agitated and aggressive. His mother had just explained that they could not do something he'd wanted to do until the following week and he was repetitively asking why and becoming progressively louder and moving toward her in a physically

threatening manner. Together, his mother and I worked to regulate him, offering physical calming strategies including a back massage from his mother. We named his feelings and empathized, before noticing that his thinking was stuck, so we returned to an activity we had completed previously around this (the *Washing machine*, see Chapter 5). As the session progressed, we moved into naming some of the things he was upset by while using physical activities that supported him to calm his body, providing play activities that supported him to calm his body. At various points in the session he needed to take a break and was supported to walk out into the hallway where he kicked a soft ball before returning to the room when he was ready to do so.

One of the aspects that we often consider in working with children is whether we need to begin with a top-down or a bottom-up approach. A top-down approach to therapy begins with the topmost areas of the brain: it focuses on what children say, how they think, and what they tell us about how they are feeling. For example, cognitive behavioral therapy is an example of a top-down therapy. In contrast a bottom-up approach begins with feelings and sensations, those which occur in the lower parts of the brain such as the brainstem and limbic system.

The way in which children talk about their feelings often helps us understand which sort of approach might work best for them because top-down strategies are very much language-based. For example, is the child able to reflect on what triggers their anger and how it feels when their anger starts to build? Are they able to describe how they can look after themselves when they are angry or what they might do to regulate themselves?

Children will often have some language around their anger; however, it is important to consider this carefully. For example, some children will be able to list strategies, such as taking a breath or walking away, despite not using these in practice. This sort of response seems to indicate that top-down strategies have been encouraged without a clear recognition of where the child is at. Your observations of the child if they have become dysregulated in those first sessions, or descriptions of what actually happens in those moments, are a more useful guide as to where to start with a child. Delahooke (2020) rightly points out that most children are assumed to be making choices when angry, though in reality they are so dysregulated at the time that they are unable to make conscious choices.

When children find it difficult to use language to talk about their feelings and experiences, we often need to use more bottom-up strategies. Supporting grownups to co-regulate their child is a bottom-up approach. The experience of having their emotions named as they experience them gradually helps them build a language around feelings and can help them engage more with top-down strategies over time. Non-directive therapies such as child-centered play therapy can be particularly helpful for these children, as can naming these emotions as they occur in sessions. Environmental adaptation is also a key approach with children and fits in the bottom-up category; reducing triggers and stressors is often one of the simplest things to start with in therapy.

It is also important to note that some children are dysregulated so much of the time that it is best to start with bottom-up strategies, such as helping them to develop safe and positive relationships and identifying and reducing their triggers. Once they are more regulated, they (and their grownups) are often in a better position to notice shifts in regulation and be able to work through these together. Furthermore, bottom-up regulation strategies, such as creating safety and ensuring the body is nurtured with good food, physical activity and sleep, can have a big impact on a child's ability to regulate their emotions throughout the day. Exploring family rhythms and identifying any of these areas that need to be considered is incredibly worthwhile.

In many ways the idea of working bottom-up or top-down is a false binary: both approaches are important and therapy is never purely one or the other (Delahooke 2020). Instead we move back and forth between the two, often doing so within the same session, as described in the example above of Levi. We may also move from focusing primarily on bottom-up to a top-down approach as our work with a family progresses, as in the example of Heidi. Even when a child is able to engage in cognitive (top-down) approaches, we need to remain attuned to non-verbal cues as we relate to them and constantly work to create safety within our relationship.

Play is a unique medium, which offers both a bottom-up and top-down experience and allows a child to integrate the two in real time (Delahooke 2020). The natural regulation that occurs when children play provides a bottom-up experience and allows the therapist to create cycles of up and down regulation, helping the child's nervous system to begin to move more readily in and out of different states. The use of symbols in play, however, also helps the child to put language to their experience, drawing out subconscious thoughts and feelings and supporting top-down thinking (Delahooke 2020).

For example, the *Washing machine* activity in this book was created when I had a child in my session who was very angry about something and was repetitively cycling back to this. She utilized some of the sensory items in the room, while her mother and I named her feelings. Her mother was able to add some calming touch at times too, and these bottom-up strategies helped her experience some regulation, settling her body briefly; however, she quickly returned to expressing her anger at not being able to do what she wanted. Straddling that space between top-down and bottom-up strategies, I gently observed that she seemed a bit stuck, a bit like a washing machine that kept going round and round washing the clothes without moving on to draining. She smiled when I said this, letting me know that I had understood the experience for her. I encouraged her to use her body to make a motion of what a washing machine stuck on a wash cycle might look like and we ended up all making our own washing machine motions, which created more smiling and laughing. The language we were able to put to her experience (top-down) as we moved our bodies (bottom-up) allowed us to have moments of co-regulation, in which we collectively spun our hands to signify the washing machine going around and around. She was able to move into a space of regulation, and the washing machine pattern became something that her family could notice and name for her outside of sessions.

Working within the zone

SAMIRA

In getting to know Samira during our first sessions I realized that she struggled to notice and name her feelings. She also appeared uncomfortable when I tentatively guessed at her feelings and was adamant that she never got angry despite her parents describing significant outbursts. Samira's parents were looking for strategies that she could use to calm herself when angry; however, I was aware that this was going to be far too complex for Samira given her current level of emotional awareness. We talked about working toward Samira being able to calm herself, noting that the first steps would be for Samira to develop greater awareness of her own feelings and for her parents to be better able to soothe her when she was becoming dysregulated. I also suggested that we explore a bit more about Samira's recent transition to school and learn how she was managing there with the understanding that we might explore further assessment as needed.

In therapy we meet the child within their zone of proximal development. Vygotsky (1954/1986) first described this, noting that children are able to do more when working in collaboration with a more skilled partner than they are able to do on their own, referring to this as the zone of proximal development. What this means is that with our support a child is able to learn more about anger, develop better coping strategies, and understand the role of thoughts in a way that they cannot on their own. Fuggle, Dunsmuir and Curry (2013) note that in CBT we create a zone of proximal development, collaborating and scaffolding children so that they are able to learn new ways of thinking.

Equally important, however, is that we are not trying to teach a child something that is well out of their reach. Rather, it is about finding that space in which we can stretch a child, knowing that doing so will help them to grow, without trying to teach them something they are not yet ready for. When we try to teach children something they are not yet ready for they tend to lose attention and disengage. Other children, particularly those who are keen to please, may learn the skill academically but lack any real understanding of it and be unable to put it into practice in their day-to-day lives. Sometimes, for example, these children will be able to list all of the things they should do when they feel dysregulated but not be able to actually put this into practice.

This is the other side of scaffolding in therapy. Recognizing that we are providing support and enabling a child to do more than they can on their own helps us recognize that we also need to provide scaffolding in the child's day-to-day life if they are to use what they learn in therapy in other contexts. Fuggle *et al.* (2013) note that children may need more support to generalize their ideas and skills learnt in therapy than to learn new ideas in the supported-therapy context.

It is also important to recognize that at times the scaffolding we provide in therapy and the safety of the space we create does indeed make it less likely that we will see anger in our sessions. Our skill as therapists should not be in providing an environment that is so supportive and scaffolded that children never get emotional, rather our skill is in creating a balance of safety and challenge. It's about creating a space in which children feel supported when their emotions get too big—a space in which they can learn a new way of engaging with their feelings.

Pacing therapy when children struggle to talk about their feelings

Another important consideration is the pace at which a child can engage in therapy. Children who are well supported and already have some language around their feelings and some helpful coping strategies tend to move more quickly through the therapy process. Those who lack a language around their emotions often move more slowly, needing lots of practice both in sessions and in their day-to-day lives with the support of their grownups to connect with their feelings. Children who struggle to talk about their emotions because of the uncomfortable feelings that arise when they do so also tend to move more slowly, needing us to titrate our approach so that they are able to gradually feel safer talking about these feelings. Some children, particularly those who are neurodiverse or have learning challenges, will need more opportunities for repetition and practice.

Providing lots of choice about how a child might be able to talk about their feelings often helps. For example, when a child is struggling to tell me about something, I will suggest that they try showing me and will suggest a few options for doing so, such as using the sandtray, the puppets or drawing. If talking is the child's preferred medium, you can allow them to choose how long they talk about something. For example, you can empathize with how hard it is to talk about anger and agree together that you might be able to talk about it for just one or two minutes, allowing the child to choose. It's a helpful way of engaging children who feel uncomfortable talking about this and helps them to titrate this experience and gradually begin to feel more comfortable talking about these feelings. Narrative approaches, such as talking about characters in stories who have angry feelings, can also be useful for children who are reluctant to talk about their anger, allowing them a bit of distance from this. Other options include working with the grownup in this context before engaging in child work, supporting them to notice and name the child's feelings, or you might suggest a non-directive approach to enable the child to gradually begin noticing their feelings.

Understanding what the grownups need
Holding the holders

How we care for grownups should ideally mirror the way in which we are encouraging them to care for their children. It is through our acceptance of, and empathy for, grownups that we create a safe space for them in therapy. Goodyear-Brown (2021) refers to this as the Cascade of Care in which we pour into the grownup what we want them to pour into the child. Giving grownups large doses of what you want them to give their children helps them to feel safe and supported in the therapy context: feeling understood and deeply heard. Similarly, Hughs, Golding and Hudson (2019) promote the PACE model, in which the focus is on adopting an attitude of playfulness, acceptance, curiosity and empathy, when interacting with the child and with the grownup. Encouraging grownups to use this stance with their child, the authors note that experiencing this is far more impactful than simply learning about it.

Emotionally holding the grownups so they can emotionally hold their child is an essential part of the work that child therapists do. It is particularly important when we reflect on how hopeless and overwrought many grownups are by the time they are able to access support for their children. So much of the work that we do with children relies heavily on the presence of a supportive grownup, so ensuring that we build a strong therapeutic relationship with grownups as well as children is essential.

While some grownups will readily develop a helpful relationship with you, others will take longer to do so. For some, their experience of supportive relationships may be limited, and you may need to be particularly mindful of creating safety for them, moving slowly and gently and prioritizing the therapeutic relationship throughout. For some grownups, the experience of having a positive relationship with the therapist is particularly valuable, providing a template where one has been lacking, and allowing them to utilize what they experience in their relationship with their child.

Being mindful of the level of support needed

JASON

Jason was reflecting on what had been helpful about coming to therapy with his son Max. He had been working alongside the therapist for six months or so, and it was clear that he had become much more attuned and empathetic toward Max. Jason provided Max with much more positive attention than previously and was able to engage in play. He gave direction appropriately and responded empathetically when Max became angry, engaging in calming strategies. Despite this progress, Jason struggled to articulate what he was doing differently and simply reflected that seeing the therapist interact with Max and having her provide gentle coaching in the moment had helped him to develop these skills. For Jason this was the key difference between working with this therapist and previous therapy, in which he had discussed parent-management strategies with the therapist.

First sessions help us to collaborate with grownups about their needs and consider how they might best engage in the therapy process. For some grownups, observing different ways in which they can interact with their child, having suggestions in the moment and being offered gentle feedback, can be particularly helpful. For others, being able to see and have this experience in the room with a therapist makes a big difference: talking about what they might do is not enough, they need to see what you are talking about.

Sometimes the challenge of learning a new way or walking a new path arises because a grownup has had a very different experience of being parented themselves. They may have well-established ways of relating to others and may find it hard to understand strategies such as emotion coaching and integrate these into their interactions with their child. For a grownup whose experience of childhood has been very different, which may indeed have been one of trauma and neglect, there may be nothing to base these strategies on. They lack a template to guide them and, in the absence of this, it is not surprising that they are unable to utilize the strategies therapists suggest.

The experience of parenting itself can also be traumatic. Having a child who is very dysregulated and engages in incredibly challenging behaviors when angry can be intensely distressing for grownups. Other experiences that a child may have, such as requiring significant medical intervention or being involved in an accident, being excluded by their peers or having to endure a significant separation can all be incredibly difficult for the grownups. Experiences such as these can disrupt the parenting process and often leave grownups feeling unsure of how they can best support their child. Grownups may need support to work through these experiences, either in your session or, if more appropriate, with the support of an adult therapist.

Grownups vary too in their emotional awareness. Some will readily tune in to their own feelings and those of their child, while others will find this much more challenging. When grownups struggle with emotional awareness they can find it hard to regulate their own emotions and to respond supportively when their child is emotional (Havighurst and Keogh 2017). Again, developing an understanding of this from our first sessions with a family is essential. A grownup's awareness of their child's emotions often develops through the process of having a therapist notice and name the child's emotions in sessions. Having structures that support this, such as encouraging families to have a daily check-in ritual in which everyone in the family names how they are feeling, can also help. Some grownups also find that they need to rely more on thinking about their child's experience, rather than reading their child's cues in the moment. I find that encouraging open communication allows us to best support families in this space. Some grownups find it helpful to explore why they have the challenges they do, which might involve doing some work of their own with a therapist or even exploring whether their challenge is more generally about knowing how others are feeling, which may prompt further exploration or assessment.

When working to increase a grownup's awareness of their child's emotions, there is often a parallel increase in the grownup's awareness of their own emotions (Havighurst and Keogh 2017). Many grownups engaged in therapy comment on this experience, and sometimes this reciprocal development occurs with very little overt focus from us as therapists. As therapists, however, it is also essential that we create space for exploring a grownup's emotional awareness and regulation whenever we need to do so. Havighurst and Keogh (2017) note that focusing on a grownup's awareness of their own emotions and their emotional regulation enhances our work with families. In practice, we need to be able to talk with grownups about the thoughts and feelings that come up for them when their children express big feelings like anger. We need to be able to support them to use regulating strategies as needed so they can regulate their child. It is also helpful when we can identify family factors that are adding to the dysregulation, such as excessive busyness or a chaotic home environment. Where a grownup's own mental health is a factor underlying their dysregulation, providing appropriate referrals is essential. It is also worth considering the role of individual therapy for grownups who have complex feelings around anger that relate to their own childhood experiences where these require greater exploration or support than your context allows.

It is important to acknowledge that as grownups have often responded in a particular way for a long time, they often need a lot of support to do things differently. Consider, for example, the way you use technology. In my forties at the time of writing this, I am clearly not a technological native. My teenage son has found the number of times I've had to ask him to show me how to take a screenshot on my smartphone frustrating; however, having him verbally tell me the buttons to use invariably ended in failure. I could not readily identify the buttons he was talking about, and the whole instruction became jumbled in my mind. The result was that I would often end up pleading that I was time-poor and asking him to do it for me. I'm embarrassed to recall the number of times I needed to practice this before I became able to copy the sequence of buttons and what was initially a clumsy, very conscious process, became automatic. And so it is with some grownups. Being in the clinic room and watching you engage their child in play, remaining attuned and regulating them as needed, can be invaluable. Through watching you and having your gentle guidance as they interact with their child, parents like Jason can learn different ways of being with their children. It is with kindness that we need to hold this space for grownups, remembering that new paths take a long time to develop.

Other grownups don't require this kind of support. They may be able to generate thoughtful ways of responding once they have better understood their child's challenges, without needing any suggestions. Still others will seek guidance around suggestions and will take these ideas and readily put them into practice, adapting them as needed for their individual child. Some grownups have greater resources and more time available to put in place what they learn in therapy, whereas others are just getting through the week and have little space to try something different. Again, getting a sense of this in the first sessions can be helpful and ensures we are able to work well with grownups, meeting them where they are at.

Considering the type of support needed and identifying barriers

CASEY

Casey (10 years) was extremely active and impulsive when she presented for therapy. Emotionally, she would react quickly to small triggers and was having frequent conflict with her father, who struggled to reflect on how Casey was feeling and tended to be quite reactive. They rarely had positive interactions and had been unable to talk about the challenges without shouting at each other. Both Casey and her father identified that they wanted to argue less; however, they had been unable to find a way to do so. Casey could only be briefly engaged in the room due to her high activity level and distractibility, and her father struggled to think about how he could support her differently. Given the longstanding concerns around Casey's hyperactivity and inattention I suggested the family consult with a pediatrician and explore whether Casey may have ADHD. Casey was diagnosed with ADHD and commenced medication. She was more able to engage in sessions and we were able to begin building on her calming skills. At home Casey was noted to be a little less impulsive when she became dysregulated, and her father was able to begin offering some body-calming strategies in these moments. Her father also began to notice that he too had some challenges with attention and began to work with the therapist around having a bit more predictability at home, which Casey found helpful.

In addition to considering a grownup's internal resources and learning preferences, practical considerations are also important. Whether or not a family is able to access therapy sessions consistently is a key consideration, as is whether grownups have the time and internal resources to put recommendations in place at home. The severity of a child's difficulties and the way these impact on the family are other important considerations. Families who have been struggling with significant challenges for a long period of time may feel overwhelmed and unsure where to start. Other families may need to enlist the support of family and friends or may need support from other professionals, as in the example of Casey above.

Exploring the family's goals and carefully identifying barriers to change is often helpful. Addressing barriers early in therapy allows us to work more effectively with families and reduces the likelihood that we will ask children or grownups to do things they are not yet able to do, risking the therapeutic relationship in the process. Consistent with this, Coghill *et al.* (2021) emphasize the need for person/family-centered care, which focuses on the individual's strengths and challenges as well as the child's and family's treatment goals when working with children with ADHD. Other supports that may be helpful for neurodiverse children are different therapies or the provision of funding or services such as respite care.

For other families, barriers might include being time-poor or not having the headspace to engage in therapy, having multiple other stressors or having little family support. Being aware of these challenges early in therapy allows us to consider how we can engage the family around this. Some barriers can be overcome by linking the family with other services, others are part of the family's reality, and it is important for us to hold these in mind in working with them, adjusting our expectations as needed. Other impediments are eased when the family engages in therapy and begins to see some change. Sometimes, in discussing barriers, a family might conclude that it is not the right time for them to engage in therapy after all, choosing to focus on another area before considering re-engaging. Being mindful of, and overtly discussing, barriers and impediments is therefore helpful.

Goal-setting and treatment planning

Goal-setting and treatment planning takes into account all of the above. Goals flow from the shared understanding of the problem and should be developed collaboratively. It is important to note that goal-setting goes beyond symptom reduction, focusing on the development of skills. For example, when working with children who have challenges with anger, our work is often around developing a child's ability to notice when they are becoming angry and communicate this appropriately. Well thought-out goals can also involve broader problems. For example, if a lack of attunement between the child and grownup is perceived as underlying the child's anger, their interaction may become the focus of the work.

While goals articulate the direction we are working toward with the child and family, a treatment plan is the method for which we hope to achieve these goals. Our treatment plan needs to allow for individual child considerations as well as family considerations. For example, our plan might specify the therapeutic approach we wish to take, who in the family might need to be involved and how this work might be best implemented. An example treatment plan for Marco (the boy with ADHD we met at the beginning of this chapter) is presented below.

Example treatment plan

Goals:

1. Support Giulia to better understand Marco's ADHD and how this relates to his behavior challenges.

2. Create moments of positive connection for Giulia and Marco.

3. Support Giulia and Marco to begin noticing early warning signs of dysregulation and triggers.

Plan:

1. Parent sessions with Giulia (incorporating visual learning given her stated learning style).

2. Sessions with Marco and Giulia (these will need to be play-based and involve movement to regulate and engage Marco):

   a. enabling them to engage in play and experience each other in a positive way

   b. noticing and naming early signs of dysregulation (and encouraging Giulia to continue doing so at home)

   c. beginning to notice triggers and exploring some of the stressors Marco faces throughout his day.

While treatment plans are important, we also need to hold these loosely in order to remain present with the family and their needs, which may shift as therapy progresses. We also need to be able to continually monitor how therapy is progressing, pivoting and changing plans as needed. For this reason, therapy plans, such as the one outlined above, that provide clear direction without being overly detailed or specific often work well. The following section discusses how we can track progress in therapy.

Tracking progress through ongoing assessment

LYDIA

Lydia (10 years) had been diagnosed with autism and ADHD and had frequent angry outbursts. She was very distractible in sessions, and I would often notice when her attention shifted, gently encouraging her to refocus. I would also notice when she became annoyed or frustrated, tentatively guessing at how she was feeling and offering some ways to calm her body as we began putting words to this. Her mother and I smiled broadly at each other during one session when she commented, "I'm annoyed I didn't win." It was the first time Lydia had noticed her anger building and was able to name this. It was an important sign that her ability to notice and name her emotions was beginning to improve. We were able to reflect to Lydia how impressive it was that she had noticed this.

Part of evidence-based practice requires that as therapists we need to collect data. In the context of therapy this means constantly evaluating and reviewing our progress. Therapists often assume tracking their progress requires the use of a standardized measure; however, while such measures have a place, we also need to use our clinical observation skills and elicit reports around progress.

Clinical observation is an important skill to develop and enables us to track a child's progress each time we see them. As in the example of Lydia, carefully noticing when a child does something different in a session is a valuable way of tracking your progress and ensuring that your therapy is facilitating positive changes. Doing so requires you to be fully present in the session, focusing on the process rather than simply on the content. Sharing these important observations with the grownups also enables them to see improvements and can support them to notice changes outside of the therapy session. The nature of therapy often means that I see children doing things differently in our sessions first, with these changes gradually generalizing to home and school.

Clinical observation of grownups and of how family members interact also provides a way of tracking a child's progress and evaluating whether the therapy is working. For example, if part of my formulation is that a child's behavior is being exacerbated by a parent's lack of insight into that child's internal experience, I will carefully notice how that grownup describes what has happened since our last session. When the grownup describes that they think their child has been somewhat anxious and overwhelmed as opposed to listing their behaviors, this is likely to mark the beginning of an important transition. It signifies that the grownup is moving toward developing a clearer understanding of their child's emotions and that our work together is progressing.

Similarly, if part of the formulation is around how children and their grownups are relating, then you can make clinical observations around this. I might, for example, notice when a child leans toward a grownup for physical comfort or reassurance, if this is not something that child typically does. Noticing that a child and grownup are able to laugh and have fun together in a session or noticing when they can discuss a challenge that has been occurring at home may also be relevant. Again, your formulation and goals will guide your clinical observations and enable you to track a child's progress and ensure that therapy is helping and is therefore evidence-based.

You can also ask grownups about what they are noticing to ensure that the therapy is being associated with positive improvements. For example, if you are working on encouraging a child to express their anger with words rather than by hitting out, you can check in with grownups about times when a child has been able to do so or note a decrease in the number of hitting incidents. It is important to remember that change can take time, so looking for small indicators that a shift is occurring can really help. Noticing, for example, that a child is calming more quickly than previously is a good sign that their ability to regulate is developing. Therapists who check in about progress with grownups and ask about symptoms without being attuned to these subtle indicators of change are at risk of inadvertently causing grownups to feel concerned about the progress and not give the therapy process enough of a chance.

Another way to check for improvements is to elicit the grownup's views on how therapy is progressing. Asking about what is working (and not working) from their perspective allows you to create an open dialogue and assess their satisfaction with the process. I often ask about what has been helpful and anything that has not been helpful. Asking about whether there is anything else they feel we should be doing can also be useful. These discussions position the grownups as active partners in the therapy and provide a space in which the therapist can also share their feedback and any suggestions about how the family might be able to get more out of the therapy process. This open collaboration also goes some way to establishing a good therapeutic relationship, which has been found to be associated with positive outcomes.

CHAPTER 4

CALMING THE BODY

MUHHAMED

Muhhamed was a 10-year-old boy who had been diagnosed with autism and ADHD. He had angry outbursts, which were often triggered by needing to stop gaming or being asked to do something that was not of his choosing. Muhhamed was often verbally and physically aggressive during these outbursts. His parents engaged in some therapy and began providing increased warning and structure. The therapist also supported them to explore calming techniques for Muhhamed. Muhhamed preferred to be alone when angry and learnt to take himself to his room, often calming himself by shooting hoops in his indoor basketball hoop. His parents began to wait till he had calmed before talking to Muhhamed about what had happened and were pleased to find that he could engage briefly in these conversations.

Calming the body is the first step in regulation. Logic doesn't work when children are distressed and talking doesn't help. Connecting emotionally and calming a child's body, therefore, is always the first step in emotional regulation. Siegel (2012) refers to this as "connecting with the right" (i.e. connecting with the right brain), encouraging grownups to connect with a child emotionally to regulate them.

As noted in the section on first sessions, assessing coping skills and calming strategies is essential. This helps us to identify any skills the child is already using and to build on these. It also alerts us to unhelpful strategies, which we may be able to support the child and grownups to shape into more effective strategies as we move into therapy.

Our first sessions also help us to identify resources that can be used to develop coping skills and calming strategies. For example, in learning about the family we might understand that the child's father is supportive and attuned and could be encouraged to offer some physical comfort, which we've learnt the child finds calming, in moments of dysregulation. Similarly, we might identify that the child has a supportive teacher who might be able to check in with the child after lunchtime, providing a space for reflection and ensuring the child has a break prior to returning to the classroom if need be, which may prevent the child's stress continuing to build throughout the afternoon. On the other hand, we might learn that the child's support system is very limited and stretched, which may prompt us to put other supports in place and encourage us to think realistically about the sort of support that could be provided.

With this knowledge in mind we can begin thinking about how we can best support children to develop calming skills. There are two main ways in which I introduce calming in therapy: as calming rhythms that we use proactively and as skills children can use in times of dysregulation. Each is discussed and there are a number of therapeutic activities included that allow us to explore these ideas with children and families.

Calming skills are presented here as it is often one of the most effective strategies we can offer early in therapy. Increasing a child's ability to regulate can provide some initial relief and can support the family to utilize some of the strategies shared later in this book. Ensuring the child is well supported and has some good coping strategies also helps to prepare the child and family for the emotions and challenges that may arise as they move into therapy. Ensuring a child has some well-developed coping skills is particularly important for children who have experienced trauma. Goodyear-Brown (2010) highlights the need to ensure that children are well supported and have good coping skills to draw on prior to intentionally processing trauma.

Developing calming and self-soothing routines

One of my children loves to shower, finding it soothing after a stressful day. Another needs to talk, doing so as soon as I greet them. The other likes to shoot hoops, sharing what has been challenging when I join them. I like to talk about what happened after a stressful day, sometimes calling a friend in the car on the way home. At other times I run a long hot bath for myself and spend some time reading.

Having rhythms and routines in our day that allow a child to have some calming moments is ideal. Families may already have calming rhythms, such as reading quietly or listening to a relaxation script in bed, while others will not yet have developed them. Learning about any calming rhythms in our first sessions is often helpful as it can be useful to extend upon these. Where families don't have calming rhythms in place we can use what we have learnt about the family and their resources to collaborate about what might be helpful in this space. What follows are some considerations around this.

Expressing a curiosity about the family's rhythms and routines is a good way to open up the conversation with grownups. For many families, the pace of life is frenetic, with a merry-go-round of school, work and sporting and social commitments. There is little time for calming or soothing rhythms in this context, and the awareness of a child's need for this can get lost. Sometimes opening up the discussion can lead to a renewed awareness of the need for this.

Supporting grownups to consider this from a developmental perspective is helpful. Most will appreciate that younger children need more opportunities for downtime and non-directed play, however adopting a developmental lens can help grownups to see why neurodivergent children may also benefit from more calming rhythms across their day. For example, neurodivergent children often benefit from having a good amount of downtime after school and may be very tired by the time the weekend arrives, benefiting from having fewer social commitments and more time at home.

Sometimes there is a mismatch between a child and a grownup in this space. Grownups who find social interaction energizing and enjoy a fast pace to their life may find it helpful to reflect on how this does or doesn't fit with the needs of their child. At other times a grownup's mental health may have made it difficult for them to hold their child's needs in mind, and it can be helpful to talk with the therapist about having more clearly defined rhythms or routines around mornings, mealtimes and bedtimes.

As discussed, what children find calming varies and the rhythms and routines will need to work for the individual child. For example, for children who find water calming, including a bath in their daily routine can be very regulating. For children who find exercise calming, ensuring that their sporting activities are spread over the week and allowing time for a park play on days they don't have something scheduled might be useful.

Ideally, we want to see grownups building some calming and self-soothing routines into their days too. A cup of tea and five minutes of quiet can be incredibly calming, as can the process of walking to school to pick up children. When grownups are engaging in calming and self-soothing routines themselves, they are in a far better position to regulate their children.

Calming in sessions

As noted previously, having emotions arise in the room presents a valuable opportunity. It's a great chance to co-regulate the child and build a child's ability to regulate. In this section we talk about how to build regulation skills in sessions, using both more and less directive techniques. As therapists, we are often in a good position to know when children are becoming dysregulated. We typically understand their triggers and can read their early warning signs. This enables us to support children through these experiences and help them to have a different experience.

It's helpful to get a sense of what a child's day has been like so far as you begin a session. This allows you to appreciate how far you might be able to stretch a child in the session, using this and your knowledge of them to find a space in which emotions can be brought into the room whilst still finding a balance and keeping the child just within their window of tolerance. For example, if I know a child has had a really hard morning and I am aware that competitive games are often a trigger for them, I'm likely to suggest something simpler. I might suggest that we play a cooperative game in which we are both on the same side and there is less intensity around winning. Doing so might allow the child to still practice regulation though will reduce the intensity and hopefully keep the child within their window of tolerance.

Another strategy that is useful within sessions is to anticipate when something might be challenging for a child. Having done so, flagging how the child might be able to manage the challenge is often very helpful. For example, you might say something like "Playing games can be tricky. I know I sometimes get frustrated. If either of us gets annoyed today when we are playing, we can use the fidget toys, take a breath or even take a break until we are ready to talk about it or keep playing." These few sentences forewarn the child about the emotional experience and help them to identify some calming strategies within the room and session. Having options available in your session is important. Children might, for example, gravitate toward sensory toys or experiences, such as playing with sand, might move into a physical activity, such as jumping rope or shooting a basketball, or might need some isolation or movement, such as moving into a small tent or going for a walk. This warning is often useful for grownups too, assisting them in identifying what they might be able to do that helps.

Getting comfortable with uncomfortable feelings and thoughts is an activity (Chapter 5) that is useful in this space. It prompts children to prepare for doing something uncomfortable in the sessions. This might be talking about something that made them angry or doing something they find frustrating. When we ask children to do something that we know is hard for them, it is important that we help them to understand why this is likely to be helpful. Sometimes this is about knowing that we don't want to miss out on the positive elements of this experience, that these things get easier over time, or that it's important to be able to do the uncomfortable thing.

During the session we can then notice any early signs that the child is becoming dysregulated, gently naming these and offering a calming strategy. For example, we may say something like "That roll really didn't go how you wanted. That was annoying." We might also offer a calming strategy. For example, we might say something like "I wonder if we should take a break" or "Maybe you, Grandma, and I should stomp out our annoyed feelings." These opportunities for in-the-moment regulation can be incredibly powerful, offering the child a chance to experience co-regulation.

It is important that regulation in the session is not about extinguishing or stopping the feeling. Rather, it is about being with the child and connecting to the emotion. It is about creating safety and giving the child space and time rather than hurrying them through. This may mean that the focus of your session shifts and becomes on regulation. Regulation is a core component of our work rather than simply something that gets in the way of what we planned to do in a session.

Calming and coping strategies for day-to-day life

MARK

Mark (10 years) was struggling with angry outbursts at home. He would often shout and hit out at his mother, Sue, when angry. Sue would become quite dysregulated in response and would say some very upsetting things to him in this context, which in turn further angered Mark. It would take a long time for them both to calm, and Sue would feel very guilty after these interactions, often berating herself about what she "should be" doing instead. Mark's narrative about how he dealt with challenges was shaped by Sue's comments, and this made it more difficult for him to see that he could respond differently.

Calming strategies and coping skills are not a magical cure; however, they are an important first step. Having some ways of calming helps children to look after themselves when they are dysregulated and ensures that they don't make the problem worse. By the time families come to therapy, the lack of regulation means that they are often engaging in ways that make the problem worse. As in the example of Mark above, this is often true both in the short term and the longer term. Sue's tendency to become dysregulated herself meant that she wasn't able to calm Mark in the moment, and these interactions impacted on how they saw themselves and each other, shaping their relationship in the longer term.

Dialectical behavior therapy (DBT) was initially developed by Marsha Linehan whose colleagues, Rathus and Miller (2015), went on to develop a manual for using this approach with adolescents. In DBT there is a strong focus on distress-management skills. Rather than being intended to resolve issues or even to shift a child's or grownup's mood significantly, these skills are aimed at ensuring that children and grownups don't respond in a way that makes the problem worse. These skills are therefore seen as a starting point, rather than an end point. For example, in the situation with Mark above, ensuring that the family can use some calming options is likely to decrease the sequelae of problematic interactions.

There are some important implications that stem from this. First, calming activities will not necessarily be enjoyable. To be effective, calming options need not bring the child joy, rather they simply need to prevent the child from aggravating the situation. The aim is not to take away the feeling, but to prevent the child from acting on that feeling in a way that makes the situation worse. A child's anger is informative, telling us about what is important to them and what might need to change. For this reason, we don't want to take away the feeling, instead we want them to be able to think about what the feeling is telling them and make a conscious choice about how to respond to this. Therefore, the aim of a calming activity is to regulate the child so that they can reflect on their anger and choose how they respond.

This is important to keep in mind when thinking with children and grownups about which calming activities have worked and which haven't. A child who has been able to use breathing to regulate themselves but still very much feels angry about a situation might reflect that it "didn't work" because they have an expectation that the breathing would result in them feeling better. If, however, the breathing prevented them from lashing out in anger and has allowed them to choose instead to let a teacher know about the situation, we would consider this as very much having worked. The calming strategy has allowed them to make a considered choice about how to respond to their feelings. This is particularly important to keep in mind when children choose a calming activity that they generally find pleasurable. For example, a child who loves listening to music may choose to try this as a calming strategy, expecting that it may bring an elevation of feelings the way it typically does when they do so. Ensuring that children are aware that the aim is not to decrease the feeling, though rather to avoid acting on it in an impulsive way, is crucial here.

Communicating with children and grownups that calming strategies are about putting us in a space where we can connect to our feelings and make good choices about these is helpful.

Increasing calming strategies

Having a repertoire of coping skills means that children are better placed to manage when difficult things happen. Being able to draw on a range of skills will mean that children are more likely to be able to find something that suits their individual situation. Hence, we often try to build upon a child's coping strategies and add to their repertoire.

Different children respond to different strategies so we need to help them explore what works for the individual child rather than prescribing a limited set of calming strategies. Lots of children will respond to physical comfort from their grownups; however, others will find being on their own more calming. Children might need calming strategies that are different from those that their siblings find helpful and are likely to need strategies that are different to those their grownups employ. Being curious and exploring a broad range of calming strategies is useful. Occupational therapists are particularly helpful in this space, using their knowledge of the child's sensory preferences to offer options that work particularly well for this.

The box below includes some ideas that you can explore with a child in your therapy room or encourage them to try with their grownups at home.

Body calming ideas for children

Jumping on a trampoline

Shooting hoops or hitting a ball against a wall

Dancing

Having a warm drink

Having a cold drink

Sinking into a bean bag

Having a shower

Splashing cold water on your face

Having a shoulder massage

Rocking in a rocking chair

Making calming tools, such as stress balls and bath bombs, in sessions with a child is often helpful. It allows you to talk about the things that they find challenging and how they can look after themselves in these situations. You can think about how they might be able to use the tool you make together and where they might keep it. Grownups can be encouraged to think about how they can support children to use their tools. A list of tools that can be made in session with children is provided below.

Calming tools you can make with children

Stress balls with various fillings, depending on the child's preferences (e.g., Play-Doh, rice, sand)

Scented handkerchiefs (scent with essential oils or other smells)

Notebooks covered with fabric that the child finds calming (e.g., silks, fluffy material or sequins)

A box or pouch of small sheets of bubble wrap to be popped

Drink bottles with words or pictures that elicit coping strategies

Screensavers for computers or tablets with pictures that are associated with calm feelings for the child

A playlist for their phone that they identify as calming

The best way to explore which calming strategies work is to encourage grownups and children to notice what happens when they try a calming strategy. You can ask about what happens when they try a specific strategy, encouraging children to notice what happens in their body as well as their feelings and thoughts. For many children and grownups, this sort of noticing can be quite new, so doing this in sessions is likely to be very helpful. When you notice that a child is becoming dysregulated, you can offer a calming strategy, such as a fidget toy, and notice any changes you see as they try it. Encouraging the grownup to also notice these changes and to reflect on whether they themselves need something to support them to regulate is often helpful.

Pit stops

This activity is helpful for exploring when children might need a break. It's a useful way to help children and their grownups think about calming rhythms.

What you need
Toy cars and either a sandtray or a large piece of paper and some markers.

Introducing this activity
When introducing this activity, you can ask about whether the child has ever seen car races on television. Ask about their experience of watching this and what they know about pit stops. Explain that pit stops are a chance to refuel and repair, making sure that the car is ready to keep driving. You can encourage the child to create a track in the sand or draw one on the paper so that they are able to drive the cars around. Talk with the child about where the pit stops need to be and include these on the track.

When the child is familiar with the idea of the cars stopping to refuel, you can explain that people need pit stops too. I often say that we all get tired and overwhelmed at times, which makes it harder for us to manage challenges and increases the likelihood that we will make poor choices when we are angry. You can then prompt the child and their grownups to consider the following questions:

- How do you know when you need a pit stop?

- In what ways might your body let you know it's time for a break?

- What is the best way for you to refuel?

- What is it that helps you feel calm and ready to deal with challenges again?

- Are you someone who can refuel quickly or do you need longer?

You can use some indirect teaching here by sharing about how you know you need a pit stop and what helps to refuel you. Grownups can also be encouraged to share about their own need for breaks. Older children are often able to reflect on many of these questions for themselves, though younger children will rely more on their grownups.

Considerations and adaptations
The conversations you have around this activity can be varied depending on the needs of the family. Sometimes this can elicit a helpful conversation about what might happen when both the child and the grownup are on their last laps and in need of a pit stop. Or you might be able to notice that when the grownup is well fueled, they are more able to support the child to have a pit stop. Sometimes this can be a good opportunity to reflect on how much energy it takes a child to drive the track, noticing that they need more frequent and longer pit stops. This is particularly true for children who are neurodiverse, and it often requires some adjustment from their grownups.

The activity provides a good opportunity to think about the need for sleep, regular meals, exercise and downtime. While these may seem like obvious needs that most families readily consider, they can get lost in the busyness of family life, particularly when families are struggling with emotional challenges, so this is worth exploring with the family if relevant.

Following the activity, you might ask the family to notice their pit stops or see if they can build in an additional pit stop during the day. The family might like to take a photo of the cars in the sand or they could take the large sheet of paper with them as a reminder of the discussion. Alternatively, older children might like to draw themselves as a car as a reminder of the need to refuel.

If you are working online and the child has a toy car at home, you can encourage them to create a track for this. Older children might be engaged through drawing a racing car online.

Calming animal shapes

This is a useful activity for beginning to work on co-regulation. It is particularly appealing for young children and is a useful way of starting to engage grownups in the process of co-regulation.

What you need
The child and one of their grownups.

Introducing this activity

The activity involves having the child make different animal shapes and exploring which of these they find calming. I begin by asking the child about any animals they know about and encourage them to think about the shape the animal makes. I invite the child to make the shape with their own body and explore whether they find it calming. For example, children may want to curl up in a tight ball like a hedgehog or echidna, or pull their legs in tight and tuck their head in like a turtle. As we notice the shapes they make with their bodies we can wonder about whether there are any animal shapes that might help when they have feelings such as worry or anger. You can play around with some ideas in the session, having the child try these out and consider what works for them.

Grownups can be encouraged to use this activity to support their child through the emotion. For example, you might suggest that the grownup might like to trace some spikes on their child's back if they are trying out the hedgehog/echidna shape, gently talking in a low volume as they do so. Similarly, a grownup might trace a shell pattern on the back of a child who is trying out a turtle shape. A baby kangaroo is another good animal shape to try with a child coming close to a grownup and being enveloped in their arms as a cozy pouch. Having this sort of direction in the play can be helpful for grownups for whom the experience of offering physical comfort is less familiar. Explaining to grownups that sometimes children need our support when they are having big feelings and that this sort of physical regulation is often the best way to begin supporting children is often helpful.

Considerations and adaptations
In encouraging grownups to use some touch, it is important to ensure that they remain attuned to their child. For those grownups who find this more challenging, you might gently help them to notice, for example, how a child responds to their touch, withdrawing or modifying this as needed. Supporting grownups to check in with children around the touch is also important, as is providing a space for grownups to talk about what this is like for them if they appear to become triggered. This activity may not be a good fit for older children, particularly if they have begun to feel self-conscious about being hugged by their grownups, so do be alert to this. It is also important to consider children who do not like touch or are triggered by touch. These children might be happy to make animal shapes without having their grownup touch them while they do so.

Talking with the family about what they noticed is often a useful reflection. You can ask about what shape worked best for them and why. You can also ask if there are times when making that animal shape at home might be helpful. Carefully noticing times of heightened emotion in your session and wondering whether the child might again want to make an animal shape is often helpful.

Taking your emotional temperature

Grownups often check their child's temperature by placing a hand upon their forehead. It is a rudimentary check, though is one that represents a moment of connection and forms the basis of this activity, which aims to support grownups to better understand how their child is feeling and to increase communication around emotions.

What you need
The child and one of their grownups.

Introducing this activity
You can begin by being curious about whether the child's grownups ever check their temperature in this manner. You may like to ask if they can show you how they do so, encouraging them to check with the child prior to placing a hand upon their forehead. Exploring the child's understanding of the process and ensuring that everyone understands this is a simple way of checking whether the child is unwell is helpful. You can then wonder about whether this process would work for feelings. Allowing some time to chat about this is often helpful, and you can then begin playing around with how grownups might check the child's emotional temperature.

The grownup might like to place their hand on the child's forehead and see if they can tell how the child is feeling emotionally. Encouraging grownups to guess and letting the child confirm whether they got this right is often fun. You might also suggest that there might be a different way to take emotional temperature and suggest the grownup try out other options, such as putting a hand to the side of a child's face or placing a hand gently on their shoulder. Children and grownups often have suggestions about how the emotional temperature could be taken and can play around with this idea. Again, encouraging the grownup to ask for consent is important here.

As the grownup takes the child's temperature and begins making guesses about how they are feeling, try to notice what they are observing about the child. Are they focusing on the child's face, for example, or tension in their muscles, or are they using their knowledge of the child? Drawing out the information sources the grownup is using and offering others as needed can support grownups to better tune in to their child's experience.

Considerations and adaptations
Because these activities are playful and fun, children will often be quite happy as they engage in this process with their grownups. This means that the process allows for positive connection; however, it does limit the range of emotions you are likely to be able to explore when you first introduce this. That said, the idea is one the family can carry through into their day-to-day life, and it is often helpful to identify a part of the day in which it would be useful to have a temperature check. For example, a family might decide that it is helpful to check the child's temperature after school and begin to do so as part of their coming home rhythm. Doing a feeling check at a time like this tends to elicit a broader range of emotions and can help the child and grownups communicate about these.

Grownups can use this knowledge of how their child is feeling to modify their expectations with a view to keeping the child within their window of tolerance. Once you have introduced this activity, you may like to encourage the child and their grownup to do an emotional temperature check at the beginning of each session.

Neurodiverse children might find this metaphor challenging, so you might like to create an emotional thermometer using craft foam or laminated cards and use that for taking their emotional temperature. Others may prefer not to be touched, so you may need to modify the activity by having the grownup either hold their hand some distance from the child's body or use the thermometer you create from a distance. Having a grownup take the child's temperature without touching is also helpful for children who find touch triggering, enabling them to engage in this activity and connect with their grownup without feeling unsafe.

This activity can also be readily completed online, though it is helpful to ensure that you can see as much of the child and grownup as possible when doing so. This will enable you to help the grownup notice any body cues that indicate a child is feeling a given way.

Breathing sensory bag

This activity supports children to notice their breathing and to understand how this can be used as a regulation strategy. Using a sensory bag for this provides children with some soothing sensory input and gives them something to focus on, which often assists them to regulate.

What you need
A clear plastic sandwich bag with a ziplock seal, some clear hair gel, a small pom-pom (0.5cm or smaller), and a permanent marker. Glitter can also be used to decorate the bag.

Introducing this activity
How you introduce this activity will depend on whether breathing is something you have used with the child before or whether you are introducing this for the first time. If you are introducing breathing for the first time, you might say something along the lines of "Breathing really helps when we start getting angry. We breathe in through our noses, fill up our lungs, and take a really loooong breath out." Modeling taking a breath in the session is important, and once you've had the child practice, you can begin talking about the shape the breath makes through your body. As you are talking, you can draw this shape with the permanent marker on the outside of the sandwich bag, explaining to the child that you are going to create a breathing bag that they can use when they need to take some deep breaths. Children are often able to reflect on the breath curling in through their nose and then slowly being released, creating a shape like the one on the next page. If they are not able to do so however, you can help them with this. Ensuring that the bottom part of the shape extends further is important as we want to encourage a longer breath out to help the child regulate.

I then squirt some clear hair gel into the bag. A couple of tablespoons is often enough, though this will vary depending on the size of your bag. Ideally, when you seal the bag you want a small layer of gel throughout the bag. Once you have squirted the gel in you can add glitter and a small pom-pom. Then try to ensure that you remove any remaining air from the bag before sealing it up. When it is sealed up, encourage the child to have a feel of the bag and explore this experience. Demonstrate that the child can gently push the pom-pom through the gel and allow them to do so.

When the child has explored the bag, I suggest that they push the pom-pom along the shape you drew earlier, breathing in and out as they do so. We then practice doing this together, slowly pushing the pom-pom around the curve as we breathe in and taking a longer breath out as we move the pom-pom along the bottom part of the shape. Grownups can be encouraged to take a turn too and may even like to create their own bag.

Considerations and adaptations
It is useful to reflect with the child and grownup about what they notice when using the bag. Talking with the child about how they might use this bag outside of sessions is also helpful. Younger children will need prompting from their grownups to use the bag while older children may be able to do this without support.

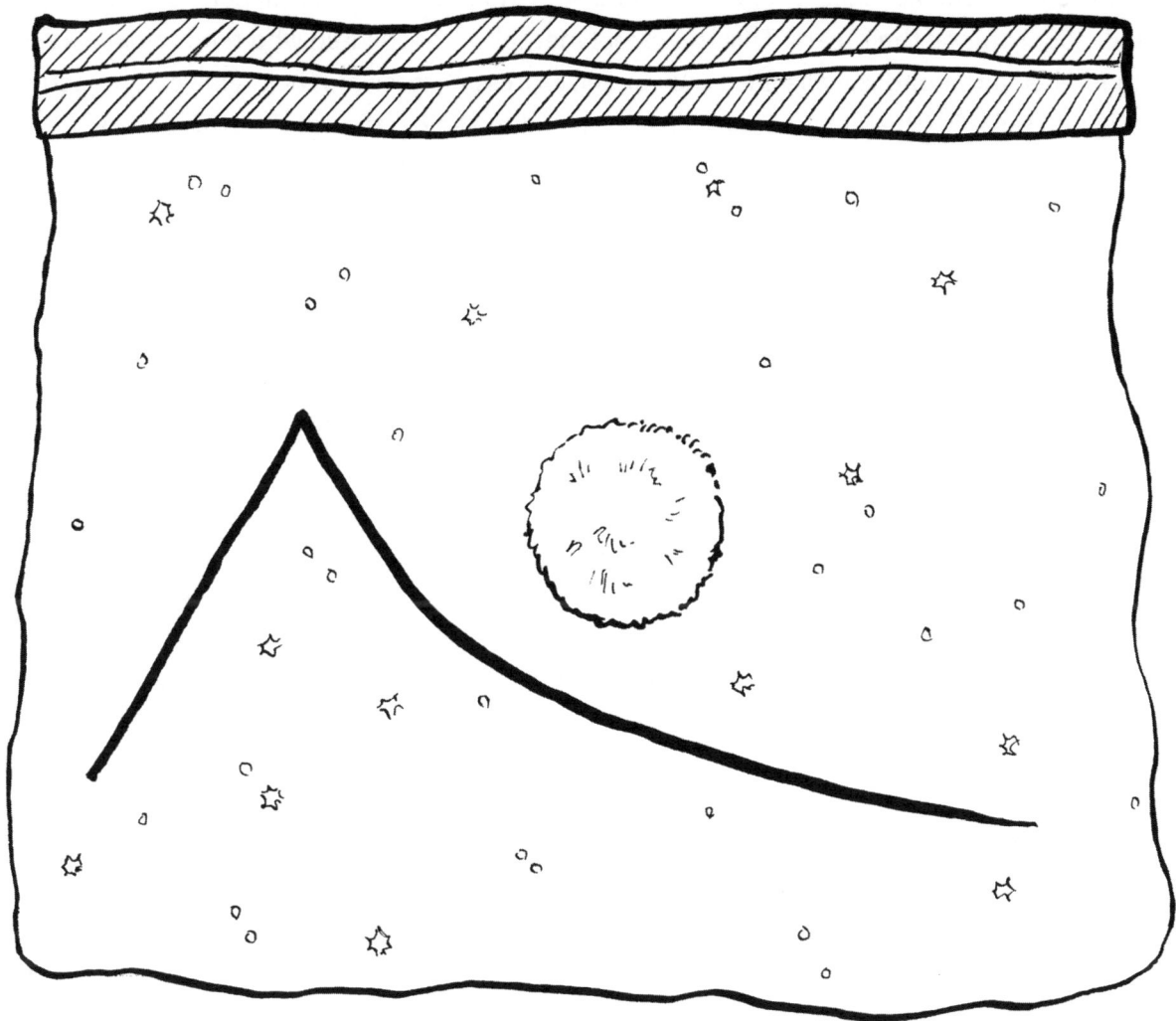

I'm on your team

Often, when we work with children around resourcing, we identify who their supports are. Sometimes we talk about this as their team. This is a useful metaphor for children who tend to have a fight reaction when angry and can misdirect their anger, expressing it toward their families. This activity helps you to talk with the family about this pattern and to begin noticing when this occurs.

What you need
Felt, scissors, craft glue and fabric markers, or the template on the next page and something to color with.

Introducing this activity
I begin by talking with the child about their team and then wonder about whether there are times when it's hard to remember this. You can then talk with the child and family about how, when things are moving quickly, it can be hard to see who is on their team, or how it can be difficult to remember who is on your team when people don't have a uniform. Encouraging the child to think about what a uniform for their team would look like and creating a jersey is often a good way to do this. Cut a jersey shape out of felt and decorate it by sticking smaller pieces of felt on it or decorating it with fabric markers. Alternatively, have a child decorate the template with markers or pencils.

While the child is making this, you can wonder together about any times that the family might have forgotten that they are on the same team and directed their anger at each other. I express curiosity about this and try to help the family to see any patterns. Wondering with the family about how they could help the child remember that they are on their child's team is also really powerful. For example, you might be able to encourage a grownup to take a deep breath and say, "I get you are angry right now. Please remember that I am on your team." Having grownups understand the misdirection of anger can also prevent them from getting caught up in responding to it and helps them instead to ground themselves and think about the child's needs.

Considerations and adaptations
The language that works will obviously vary from child to child, and it is important to ensure that grownups use less language as children become more dysregulated. Talking about when grownups might be able to use this language and what they might say is often helpful in the session, and you can reinforce this idea through some puppet play or similar.

If you are working online you can share the pdf of the jersey and allow the child to color it or ask the family to print it ahead of time so that the child can decorate it in the session.

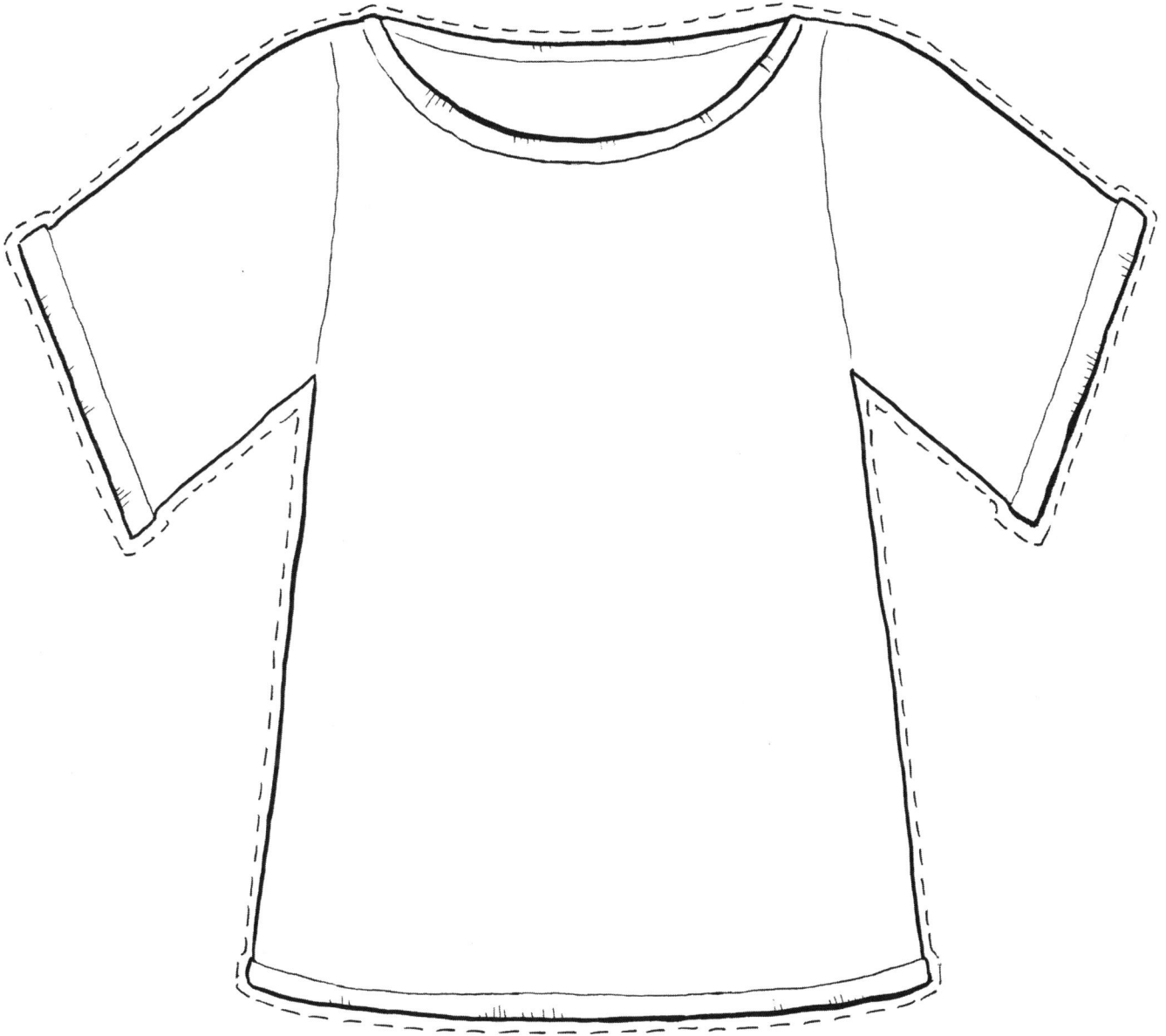

CALM for you, CALM for me

This is a useful activity for helping children and grownups reflect on their regulating strategies. It is often useful early in therapy as you begin to build upon a child's strategies, though it is also helpful later in therapy as a way to consolidate a child's coping skills.

What you need
Paper or cardboard and markers or pencils.

Introducing this activity
I introduce this activity by suggesting we see if we can find a way to think about all of the child's coping strategies and calming skills. I then explain that we could make a CALM poem, using each of the letters as a prompt to list something that helps the child to regulate. An example is included below.

Completing a poem with the child provides an invitation for them to get curious about some other strategies, and you can be mindful of this when thinking about which coping strategies you include in your poem. For example, when working with a younger child it is useful to include strategies in your poem that are appropriate to this age group, such as M for Moving closer to Mom. If you are working with an older child you can include strategies that are a better fit for them developmentally in your poem, such as L for Listening to music.

Considerations and adaptations
Younger children are likely to need more support from others to calm, so it is often worth including seeking strategies in their poems. Creating a CALM poster can work well for younger children, as this can be displayed and grownups can readily reference this when supporting a child to regulate. Older children may prefer to make a CALM card that they can transport more easily or can keep more private. Blank playing cards are good for this purpose and fit well inside a child's pocket, wallet or pencil case. Reflecting with the child and family about how they might use this outside of sessions is helpful.

Sometimes children will need support to fit their strategies to the letters of the poem. It's good to model thinking flexibly around this. For example, if a child uses help-seeking as a strategy, this could be listed under A for Ask for help, C for Call Mom, or even under M as get Mom. Those children who are particular about rules or have perfectionistic tendencies may struggle to adopt a flexible approach and may need support to explore and regulate through this. Please keep in mind that some children may have negative associations with particular words, including words such as calm, so being alert to this and choosing other words as needed is important.

This activity can readily be completed online, either using an online whiteboard or by having the child use some paper and markers at their end. Grownups can be invited to participate in this activity, creating their own CALM poem. They can also support the child to think about where they might keep the poster at home and how they might remind the child to use those strategies as needed.

Choose to take a breath

Ask for help from grownups

Look at what my anger is telling me

Move away if I need to

My magic bag

This activity is useful for helping children to reflect on their resources and identify what they can use to regulate themselves.

What you need

A brown paper lunch bag or a small plain bag. Alternatively, you can use paper or a coloring page of a backpack. You'll need markers or pencils as well.

Introducing this activity

The activity uses the concept of a magic bag, one that can store all of the resources they need. Older children who are familiar with the *Harry Potter* series may relate this to Hermione's bewitched beaded handbag in *Harry Potter and the Deathly Hallows*, in which she packs numerous resources for their mission, while younger children may recall Mary Poppins' carpet bag from the classic 1964 movie, which seems to have no bottom and is used to store large bulky items. Checking whether the child is familiar with these scenes can be a useful way of introducing this activity.

More generally, however, this activity helps children to think about the idea of preparing. When we pack a bag it is in preparation for something. We pack a towel, bathers and goggles for swimming, while we pack lunch, our pencil case and homework for school. Children often observe or are involved in packing bags throughout their week, so I often introduce this activity by getting curious about the bags they use during the week.

I then talk with children about what they would need to pack if they had a magic bag they could have with them when things get difficult, suggesting some of the situations in which I know they find it challenging to regulate. The child can then choose to make, draw or color a bag as you explore this idea. Simple bags can be created by cutting a handle into a brown paper lunch bag as shown in Figure 4.1. Alternatively, you may like to have some small plain gift bags on hand for children to decorate. Older children can be encouraged to draw a bag, particularly if drawing is an interest area or strength of theirs. Coloring in a picture of a bag is another option and you may like to allow the child to choose from some different coloring pages online. If you are working online, you could draw a bag or color a picture of one online. You could alternatively check if the family has a lunch bag you could use for this activity.

As you make, draw or color the bag talk with the child about what would go into the bag. Emphasize that this is a magical or special bag that can contain anything. Explain, for example, that you could keep a massive stop sign in it to help you remember to stop and breathe or could put a hug from a grownup in it and make something that symbolizes this.

Considerations and adaptations

When the bag has been made you might like to encourage the child to practice with it by using it in a show with puppets or dress ups. This often works well for children who need some distance from their own day-to-day challenges, though other children might be keen to role play situations in their day-to-day life, showing you how they might use the bag.

Talking with grownups about when the bag might come in helpful and what calming options they might be able to suggest from the bag is often helpful. Grownups can also be encouraged to reflect on what is in their own bags and may even like to make one of their own if they are present during the session.

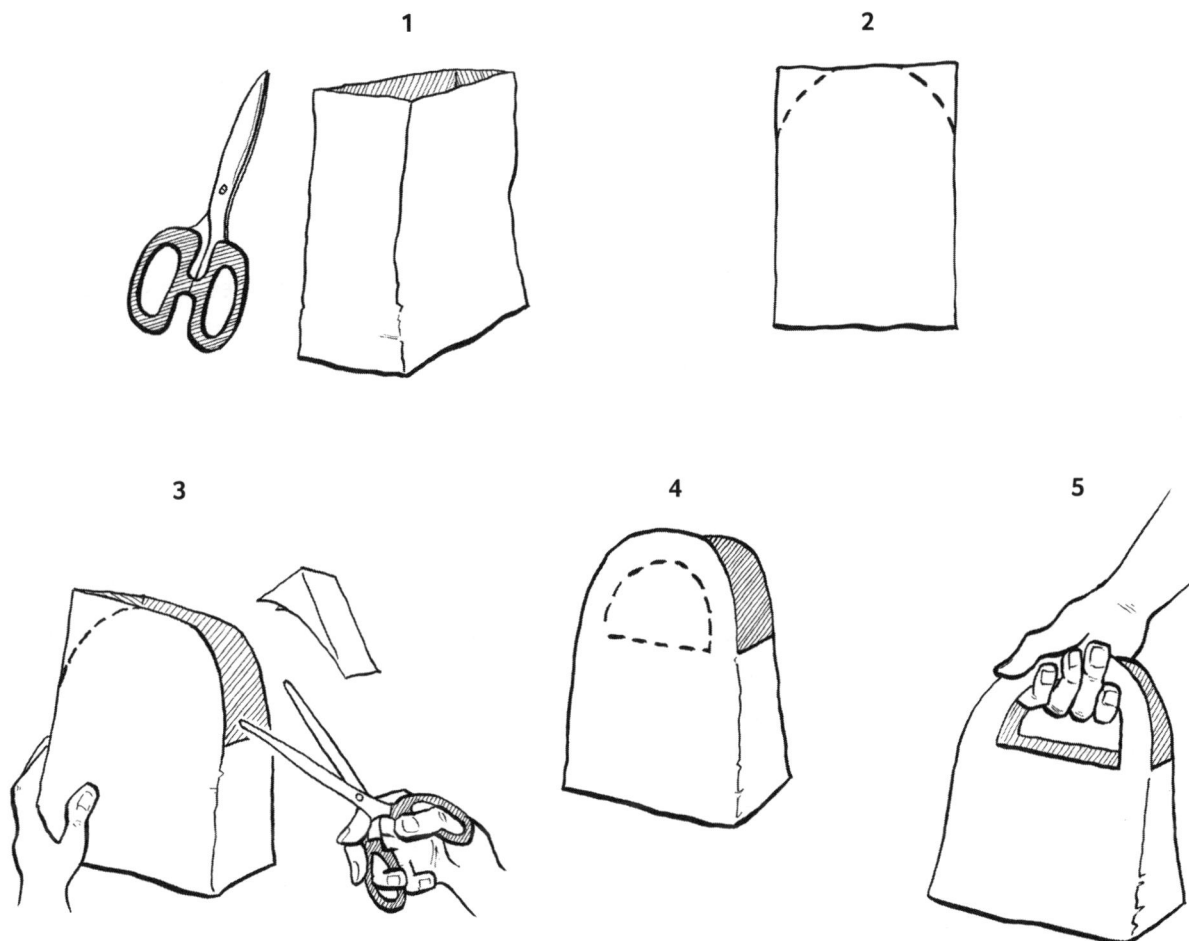

FIGURE 4.1 MAKING A MAGIC BAG FROM A BROWN PAPER LUNCH BAG

Umbrellas for angry moments

This is a useful activity for helping children and families to think about how they can look after themselves when they are angry. It works well with the *Clouds of anger* activity in Chapter 5 so you may want to think about using the two in combination.

What you need

Small party cocktail umbrellas, a toy umbrella or the template on the next page and markers or pencils to decorate it with.

Introducing this activity

Choose the materials that will work best for the child from the above list. As you color, draw or play with the umbrella you can talk with the child about what it is that an umbrella does. Umbrellas offer some protection; however, they do not stop the rain. In this way umbrellas are a good metaphor for how we can look after ourselves when we are angry. Talk with the child about the idea of anger being like rain. We don't want to stop the rain—rain is important and you can talk with the child about what would happen if it didn't rain. We can, however, look after ourselves when it rains, which is what an umbrella does, it offers some protection until the storm passes. You can share how you look after yourself when you are angry and encourage the child's grownups to share any helpful ideas they use for themselves. You can then encourage the child to think about what helps them look after themselves when they are angry. Their grownups may be able to offer some suggestions about this based on their observations, and you are also likely to have some ideas arising from your sessions. For example, you might suggest taking a big breath, cuddling with a grownup, moving their body, or remembering that the angry feeling will pass.

Depending on what works best for the child, you might choose to act out some scenarios together, practicing putting the umbrella up as you employ one of the strategies you've talked about. Some children will prefer to do this using a puppet or soft toy, identifying when the character they chose might need to pop up their umbrella, and using their breathing or taking a break rather than participating in role play themselves. Those that are able to talk through strategies may simply like to write the strategies on the umbrella they have made.

When reflecting on this activity, older children can be encouraged to think about when they might most need the coping strategies listed on their umbrella and to engage in problem-solving around how they can access these supports when they need them. For younger children and those who still require support to regulate, grownups will need to be involved in this discussion. Talk together about how they can share an umbrella with their child, encouraging them to be mindful of how they can support the child in moments of anger.

Considerations and adaptations

If you are working online, you may be able to have the child show you their own umbrella so that you can put it up and down as you speak. It's important to check with the child's grownups prior to doing this as some may not feel comfortable with the idea of doing so, and some children may need help to open and close the umbrella. You could also share the downloadable template, allowing the child to color this online if your program allows you to do so. Alternatively, some families may like to have the page emailed to them, enabling them to print it ahead of time for the child to color in the session.

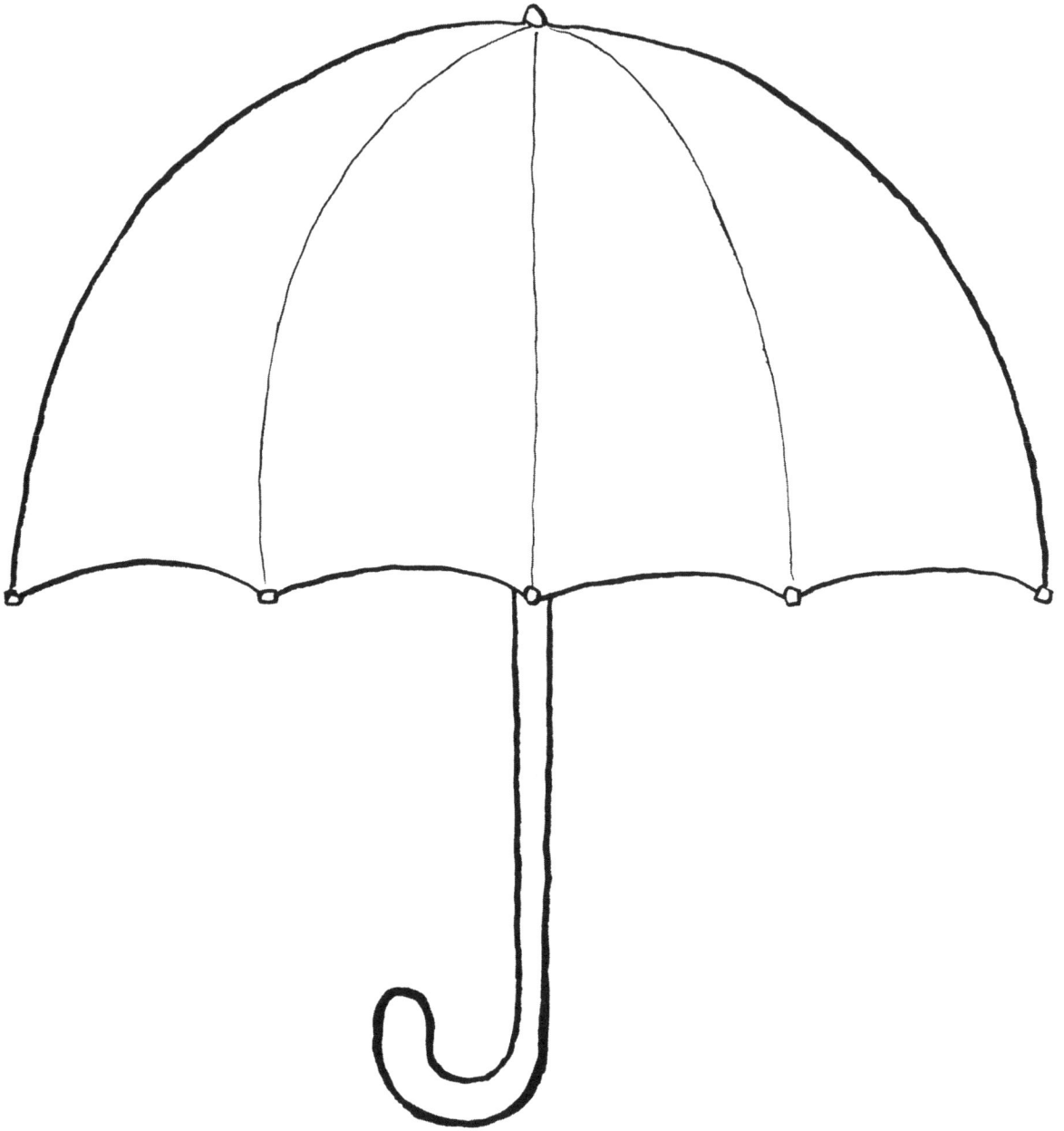

CHAPTER 5

UNDERSTANDING AND EXPRESSING ANGER

In our first sessions the focus is often on learning about the family's experience of anger. As we move into therapy, however, we often have a role in helping the family understand more about anger. As they learn more about anger, children and grownups may begin to shift the way in which they relate to this feeling. They might, for example, create space for angry feelings and begin to view these as helpful reflections and communications. Understanding is an invitation to do something differently and can therefore be an intervention in and of itself. It is also the foundation upon which intervention is built.

It is important to recognize that individual children experience anger differently. Therefore, we need to create a space in which we encourage the child and family to explore their own experiences: to lean in and get curious about this and articulate what happens for them. Often children and families have not understood their own experience of anger, and it's not something that has been discussed overtly. Using play facilitates expression (Schaefer and Drewes 2014) and supports the child and grownups to communicate far more about their anger than they would using talking alone. Understanding is a collaborative process, in which we help the family to understand a bit about anger and they help us understand more about their personal experience and come to understand it better themselves.

Implicit in this is the need to tailor our approach to individual children and their grownups. The process of understanding a child and their family and, perhaps more importantly, of supporting them to understand themselves will look different with each child and family. The way in which we explore this, the areas we focus on and the pace at which we move through this stage will all vary and will rely heavily on your clinical judgment. Choose those activities that best suit the needs of the children and families you work with and maintain a curious, accepting and empathetic stance throughout, continually checking in and evaluating your work together.

It is worth noting that the emphasis in this chapter is on understanding, rather than simply expressing, anger. Anger is complex and, as discussed, may relate to unmet needs or arise as a result of other experiences. While expressing anger is often helpful, understanding the context is essential. As therapists, we have a key role in helping the family understand both the immediate and broader context that surrounds a child's expressions of anger. This understanding helps us provide nuanced intervention, meeting the needs of the child both in the moment and more generally.

It is also worth noting that expressing anger can be helpful, particularly when doing so enables a child to connect with their grownups; however, repeatedly acting on aggressive thoughts and feelings is generally unhelpful. For example, a child who expresses their anger toward a sibling and is supported by a grownup to negotiate a compromise has an experience both of being regulated and of solving problems effectively. The child, however, who becomes stuck in their anger, expressing it repeatedly to a grownup, with lots of exclamations about how horrible their sibling is, is likely to remain angry and become stuck in a pattern of ruminating thoughts. Helping children to understand the role that rumination can play and supporting appropriate expressions of emotion that move children into action is therefore helpful. This approach fits with emerging research that suggests that angry rumination in children is associated with aggression (Harmon *et al.* 2019; Smith *et al.* 2016).

Sometimes understanding anger in and of itself is enough. Children and grownups bring their own resources, and understanding anger can be enough to allow them to put their own coping strategies and interventions in place. At other times families will continue to need support around how they might be able to manage the anger and will benefit from the ideas and activities in the chapters that follow. Either way, understanding anger is an important first step.

Finally, much in the way that assessment continues throughout therapy, facilitating understanding does not occur only at the beginning of therapy. As the foundation to our therapeutic work, our understanding of a child's anger is something that we return to often, updating it as needed. Circling back to our understanding of how the child and family experiences anger helps children and grownups understand the rationale for our other interventions and keeps our work focused.

What we want children to understand about anger

When supporting a child and their grownups to better understand their anger, it is helpful to first reflect on what it is we want them to understand about it. This section briefly introduces some of the key aspects we want children to understand about anger more broadly as well as what we want them to know about their own anger.

We want children and their grownups to understand some key points about anger, which are summarized in the downloadable handout that follows. While these points may seem obvious, they are worth exploring with families. Some families need support to remember that angry feelings will pass and can feel quite panicked when they appear. Others may need to create more space for expressing anger, while still others may need to foster appropriate expressions of anger.

Part of the therapeutic process involves helping children and grownups to better understand their own anger. Children who can recognize signs of anger in their bodies, understand their early warning signs and triggers and can effectively express how they feel are more able to manage their anger. Each of these elements is discussed further.

★

Handout: Understanding anger

Important things for children (and their grownups) to know about anger

Everyone gets angry sometimes.

Angry feelings come and go.

Anger can tell us about what is important to us.

Anger can also keep us safe.

We can be curious about our anger.

We can still make good choices when we are angry.

We can be angry without hurting others.

Recognizing anger

LUCIA
Lucia was referred for concerns around emotion regulation and was said to frequently become angry at home. She had not shared any examples of anger during our first sessions; however, her voice became louder and she looked frustrated a number of times when playing a game with her grandmother. Gently noticing her feelings in these moments and continuing to explore a range of emotions in each session, including anger, helped Lucia to begin talking about her angry feelings.

Recognizing anger is a prerequisite for many of the therapeutic strategies that follow later in the book. If a child is not aware that they are becoming angry, they are unlikely to utilize coping strategies, even if they have been taught lots of helpful techniques. As noted previously, some children will already understand what tends to make them angry and will be able to name the feeling when they experience it. Others will lack an understanding of their body signals and triggers and will need support to develop these skills.

For children in the latter category, it is necessary to focus on building their emotional awareness initially. Naming emotions in the room is really helpful in this context. For example, you might say something like "I can see that's making you angry. I'm noticing your voice is getting louder." Statements such as this provide the child with a name for what they are feeling and link this with what they are experiencing in their body, helping them to build the connection between the two. Supporting grownups to do this work is essential, as it is the repeated pairing of the emotion word with those feelings that supports the child to learn the connection. It is the empathetic stance of the grownup and therapist as they name these feelings that conveys that all emotions are ok and creates a safe space for the child to express those feelings. As the child has the experience of linking what they are experiencing in their body with a feeling word, for anger as well as all their other feelings, they often begin to label these feelings for themselves.

What is implicit in this is the need to allow emotions to come up in sessions. Emotions frequently arise in the context of play and discussion, allowing opportunities for noticing and naming. The activities in this book also often provide a structure in which emotions arise. Staying present as you complete activities and ensuring that you slow down and process these as they arise is essential.

This process is very much about emotion coaching, an approach that was initially described by John Gottman (Gottman and Declaire 1997). The approach is also consistent with the work of Siegel (2012) and the Tuning in to Kids programs.[1]

Some children quickly begin labeling their feelings when this approach is undertaken consistently, whereas for others it takes longer. Children with autism, for example, often need to spend more time developing their emotional awareness. They may express

---

1   https://tuningintokids.org.au

emotions differently, with non-verbal communication that is less typical or difficult to interpret. This can make it challenging for grownups to attune to their feelings and notice and name these, leading to challenges with co-regulation. Exploring this openly, alerting grownups to the potential for children to express emotion differently and working together to begin noticing and naming early signs both in sessions and at home is often helpful.

Recognizing how stretched the child is and seeing the build-up

Most days, I'm able to respond calmly to my children having left wet towels and clothes on the bathroom floor. I ask them to pick them up and typically this works. Some days, however, I get annoyed and grumble at them. The difference is not in the towels and clothes; generally one of my children will have left something on the floor over the course of the day at this stage in our family life. Instead the difference is within me. The days I get annoyed are the days when I'm tired and feeling stretched or have other things that have made me upset.

JEROME

Jerome was autistic and found school very stressful. Sometimes, on the way home from school, his grandmother would stop in at the supermarket to pick up items for dinner. Jerome was able to manage this some days; however, on others he would become very dysregulated and would kick the back of her car seat and shout.

MIA

Having run five minutes late to a telehealth appointment, my computer connected to show me Mia and her mother. I knew that Mia was likely to have found waiting extremely difficult, having observed her struggling with this previously and knowing that she had autism and ADHD. Mia's face showed no sign of dysregulation when I joined, and her mother readily accepted my apology. Although it had only been a small wait, I wanted to acknowledge that it had probably felt much longer for Mia and that I knew waiting was hard for her. As I took the time to do so, both Mia and her mother relaxed and were able to talk about how hard it had been. Naming the experience was regulating, and we were able to move into a regulating activity prior to doing something more challenging.

We all have an amount of stress that we can manage at any point in time. Rather than being fixed, however, the amount of stress we can manage varies. Some days, we can manage more, being able to face challenges that would be difficult for us on other days. Some days, we are already so stretched that we can manage very little and become dysregulated in response to small triggers. Our ability to manage stress can change within a given day as well: it might decrease slowly over the day in response to numerous small stressors until we feel unable to manage even one more small thing.

Children are no different. They have times when their capacity for managing challenges is far less and they can often respond in anger. This can be confusing and confronting for grownups who suddenly find their children shouting in response to small triggers. It is, therefore, really important to help both children and their grownups to understand this. Grownups who can tune in to their child, understanding how stretched they are at any point in time, are able to reduce demands and suggest calming activities that allow children to become more regulated, avoiding angry outbursts in the process.

Grownups are often juggling multiple demands, and it can be easy for them to miss signs that their child is really stretched and is reaching the edge of their window of tolerance. They might describe concerns about their child having big responses to small triggers. Grownups can feel irritated and angry, feeling that the situation did not warrant such a big reaction. This response can unfortunately be invalidating and further contribute to the difficulties the child experiences. Furthermore, it ignores what the anger might be communicating. It fails to explore what might be important to the child and fails to help the child communicate this to others. For example, a child who has a very large angry reaction to small changes of routine may be communicating that they need more support around this or would benefit from a greater level of structure. Well-meaning therapists may also be invalidating, talking with the child about how this really is a "small problem." It is important that we meet the child where they are at, acknowledging those things that are big for them, though also being curious about how stretched they might be and whether this has an impact.

Grownups can tune in to how stretched their child is both by holding an understanding of them and by tuning in to early warning signs. Holding an awareness of the child allows us to estimate how stretched they might be. As with Mia above, we can use our knowledge of children to respond to this in a helpful way, even when children aren't displaying signs that they are stressed or anxious. Grownups can also be encouraged to tune in to their child's early warning signs as a way of noticing how stretched they are. For example, Jerome's grandmother might notice changes in his body movements as he walks to the car or how heavily he closes the car door and be curious about how these changes might indicate how he is feeling. As children understand this more for themselves, some of them will begin to communicate this directly, saying things like "It's just been a really busy day" or "I'm feeling tired from school."

It is worth acknowledging here that children who have autism may have difficulty with both understanding and expressing their emotions. They may display fewer typical signs that they are becoming dysregulated, making it difficult for their grownups to read them and leading to them being perceived as going from 0 to 100 without any clear triggers. Children with autism are often less likely to communicate about their feelings, which further adds to the likelihood that they will experience an angry outburst as their stresses accumulate. It is particularly valuable to work with the grownups of these children to support them to understand the cumulative nature that this stress sometimes takes and help them to use their knowledge of their child, rather than just their early warning signs, to judge how stretched a child is.

It is important to recognize that our window of tolerance is shaped by our experiences and shifts over time. Indeed, the process of therapy often helps to stretch both the child's and grownup's windows of tolerance. While the concept is particularly helpful for trauma, it also has important implications for emotional regulation. Our window of tolerance can shift from day to day or even within a day, depending on how much we have already dealt with.

The activity *How stretched are you today?* Provides a playful way of explaining this to children and grownups using a stretchy ball and encourages them to reflect on their own regulation. I often check in at the beginning of a session to get a sense of how the child is feeling and what their day has been like up to that point. For children with whom I have introduced the idea previously, I will use the stretchy ball to help them and their grownups reflect on where they are at and relate this to how much we might be able to do in the session. As discussed previously, checking in at the beginning of a session can be particularly helpful. Increasing the amount of calming we include in a session and decreasing the demands for a child who is already very stretched is respectful and can help the child's grownup see how this might be done.

On a related note, it is helpful when we can recognize early warning signs that a child is becoming dysregulated. Noticing signs that a child is moving toward the edge of their window of tolerance allows us to pivot and provide some coping strategies or alter the environment so that they are better supported and able to move back into a state of optimum regulation. Helping children to tune in to these signs for themselves allows them to use their coping strategies sooner, allowing them to do so more successfully.

Noticing body signs

As Siegel (2020) describes, "our awareness of bodily state changes… lets us know how we feel" (p.255). The ability to tune in to our internal experiences is referred to as *interoception* and is something that we are increasingly learning more about. Helping children to tune in to their feelings remains important throughout therapy; however, knowing how you feel is also a prerequisite for much of what follows in this book and in therapy more generally. Understanding how the child notices their feelings and their ability to connect this with their bodies in our early sessions helps us understand how much or how little this will need to be the focus early in therapy.

When working to help children tune in to their bodily sensations and notice early warning signs, it is important that we engage grownups. Supporting grownups to notice bodily signs in the child's day-to-day life helps to increase the child's awareness sooner. It also helps grownups to attune more effectively to their child and supports the process of co-regulation.

Remaining focused on subtle shifts and changes throughout sessions is also very helpful in fostering a child's ability to tune in to their feelings. Pausing when you notice even subtle changes and getting curious about these helps children to better notice these shifts and allows grownups to see how they might notice shifts outside of sessions. Sharing what you notice about any of your own bodily shifts and changes during a session can also be a useful way of modeling this.

In addition you can work to build interoception through activities that focus specifically on this. Some of the activities in this chapter also encourage children to notice early warning signs as well as noticing how stress can build cumulatively over time, including *Unsafe animals, Understanding anger dice game* and *Clouds of anger*. My co-authored books *Creative Ways to Help Children Manage Anxiety* (Zandt and Barrett 2021) and *Creative Ways to Help Children Manage Big Feelings* (Zandt and Barrett 2017) include a section on noticing early warning signs in children who have anxiety, with activities that are also relevant to children who have angry outbursts.

Understanding the feelings underneath anger

As noted previously, anger is typically a secondary emotion with other emotions underneath it. Emotion-focused therapy emphasizes the therapist's role in helping to understand emotions through emotion coaching and emphasizes the importance of identifying primary emotions (Greenberg 2002). Under a child's anger, there are often other feelings, such as worry or sadness, and helping both children and grownups connect with these feelings can be incredibly powerful. Connecting with the feelings underneath a child's anger often helps us to see what the child is needing to communicate. When grownups understand the feelings underneath, they are generally able to respond far more empathetically. Activities such as *See it differently, Different feeling parts* and *Seeing the other feelings in my anger* all help children and their grownups to begin thinking about their anger in a more nuanced way, learning about the feelings that go along with or are hidden underneath their anger.

In sessions, getting curious with a child about what their angry feeling might be telling them is often a good way to explore this. You might empathize with the child about how angry they felt and wonder about whether there were any other feelings that were coming up for them. You can talk about times when you were angry and explain that part of you felt angry and part of you felt something different. You might wonder about any feelings that might be underneath their anger.

Therapists often use the iceberg analogy to explore the latter, noting that there can be a large number of feelings and stressors underneath the child's behavior. One of my favorite and simplest ways of exploring this is using an activity I outlined in *Creative Ways to Help Children Manage Big Feelings* (Zandt and Barrett 2017). In this activity, *Lift the flap on anger*, you fold a piece of cardboard to create a flap. Anger is listed on the top and as you lift the flap you begin to explore with the child the feelings that might be underneath there, writing these below. The simplicity of this activity makes the concept of there being other feelings underneath the anger very accessible for children and families and they often find this very meaningful.

When children connect with the feelings that go along with their anger, they are often more able to understand what their angry feelings might be communicating. For example, a child who can identify that they felt anxious and then angry can reflect that they may need to ask for help and could engage in a conversation about what support they might require. Activities such as *Anger word match* (Chapter 6) can help children to think about what their angry feelings might be communicating.

It is important to remember that having a curiosity about a child's anger is not the same as knowing about a child's anger. Children, grownups and therapists will not always know the reason a child is angry, even though we can reflect and have some ideas about why this might be the case. This is particularly true when children have experienced trauma and react to situations with anger as part of being triggered. Promoting curiosity does not imply that grownups, therapists or even children themselves will always know why they are angry. Rather, it encourages reflection—honoring the angry feeling, with the understanding that it may not always be clear why a child feels angry.

Having a better understanding of the feelings underneath and what the child might be communicating with their anger is also supportive for grownups. It helps them to organize their child's feelings and look for the feelings underneath when their child is angry. Being able to recognize that their child is distressed when they are angry often helps grownups respond more empathically and means that they remain more regulated, which in turn puts them in a better position to regulate their child. Chapter 6 provides a model for supporting grownups with this.

Remembering that anger will pass

Anger can often feel out of control for children and their grownups. Knowing that feelings come and go and that even very intense anger will pass eventually is often helpful. While this may seem obvious, many children and grownups don't seem to appreciate this in the moment: they get caught up trying to stop the feeling, often making things worse in the process. Having some playful ways of conveying to families that all feelings come and go can help to take the intensity out of big angry moments and enable them to navigate these more successfully.

One of my favorite ways to explore with families the idea that all feelings come and go is to use the *Feelings bubbles* activity included in *Creative Ways to Help Children Manage Big Feelings* (Zandt and Barrett 2017). It's a simple playful activity in which children and their grownups explore the idea of feelings coming and going using the metaphor of bubbles, some of which last longer and some of which pop quicker, but all of which disappear in the end. *Tunneling through the feeling* is an activity in this chapter that allows you to explore this with the family.

Recognizing patterns

Anger is expressed differently by different children: some escalate quickly, storm briefly and settle soon after; while others build slowly and take a long time to settle completely, being readily triggered and escalating again; some want to talk and shout; others stomp off and prefer to be alone. Patterns exist in families too; for example, anger might catch quickly between children and grownups, and grownups might miss the chance to try reasoning and problem-solving with children when they are dysregulated.

Helping children and families to recognize their individual patterns and curiously exploring what works well and what doesn't is important. *Getting in the tank* is an activity that helps children and families understand a child's tendency to have a fight response when angry. In a similar way the *Washing machine* activity highlights the pattern of rumination and is particularly useful for helping children who become repetitive when angry. Anger does frequently catch in families, and understanding this is often very helpful. *Creative Ways to Help Children Manage Big Feelings* (Zandt and Barrett 2017) includes an activity called *Yawn game*, in which families use yawns to explore the way in which feelings catch in families.

When anger doesn't come into the room

JULIA

Julia's parents were struggling with her angry outbursts at home. She would become verbally and physically aggressive numerous times a day, often in response to small triggers. When she met with her therapist for the first time, Julia was noted to express her feelings through her body, such as jumping up and down when she was happy. When asked directly about emotions, she was reluctant to speak about anger and denied ever feeling angry.

When therapy works well, there is often an intricate balancing of support and challenge. Sometimes the child and family navigate this for themselves, going deeper and challenging themselves more as the work progresses. At other times there is more reliance on us to find the balance, ensuring that we incorporate enough challenges to support growth while not overwhelming children and families. In the area of emotional regulation this means ensuring that there is the space to talk about dysregulation in the session. It means creating space for feelings of anger, with the understanding that having these feelings arise in the supported context of therapy enables us to support children and families through these.

For this reason, when children don't spontaneously talk about anger in a session, it can be useful to facilitate some discussion around this. Doing so is often helpful in the assessment phase, helping you understand not only what a child knows about their anger, but also giving you a sense of how they feel about it. It is also helpful throughout therapy and can be an important part of finding the balance of support and challenge. For Julia this meant gradually talking more about anger as therapy progressed. Julia was also able to move from using play and story to express anger to being able to talk directly about her anger at home. Again, this gradual shift was part of the therapy process for Julia, with the challenge gradually increasing as Julia became more comfortable expressing anger.

For those children who do not bring their anger into therapy sessions, it is important to consider the balance of support and challenge. Directly introducing some play around anger is often helpful, and a number of activities, such as *My anger song* and *Sitting with all my feelings*, can be useful in this space. Remember, though, that challenge needs to be balanced with support. If an activity becomes too much for a child, notice their response and work through it. Either modify the activity to reduce the demand, choose another activity or take a break.

My anger song

This is a useful activity for encouraging children to express anger, providing a safe space for them to do so. It is particularly helpful for children who have found it hard to express their anger.

What you need
Your singing voice and some musical instruments or a music-making app.

Introducing this activity
To introduce this activity, I notice that people make different noises when they are angry. They might for example, say *grrr* or *arrr*. I suggest that we see if we can make a song using some of these different sounds.

Children who are reluctant to express anger might feel most comfortable starting with the angry sounds and feelings of others, so you can begin with adding these into a song. For example, you might begin with something like "Grrr, grrr, grrr, when my brother feels angry, grrr, grrr, grrr, he stamps his feet." Others may prefer you to create a song first. As the child becomes more expressive, you may be able to encourage them to think more about their own experience of anger.

Creating a song, particularly a silly one, often supports a child's self-expression and allows them to share more about their experience of anger. As you develop the song, you can help them to notice what happens in their body when they get angry, noticing the sorts of sounds they might make as well as how their body might move. Indeed, some children will like to make a bit of dance as they go, which is a great way to connect in with their bodies and notice what that activation feels like.

As children create a song, you might like to help them reflect on the rhythm of the song. For example, if a child creates a fast angry song, you can wonder if that is what it is like when they are angry, with everything going really quickly. You might like to sing the song in slow motion and explore what happens when you do so.

Considerations and adaptations
Grownups can be included in this activity, being encouraged to offer suggestions and to sing along. They may also find it helpful to reflect on their own angry song and how this is similar or different to the child's. Asking the child and grownup to sing their song at the same time can be a good way to demonstrate how chaotic and overwhelming it can be when they are both angry. This activity can be completed online if the child has some instruments or an app they can use to make music.

Children might like to record a video of them singing their song or they might like to write the lyrics down so they can take these home. You can also talk with the child and grownups about how the angry song might help them recognize when the child is becoming dysregulated at home and reflect on what they might have learnt about a child's body signs or triggers.

It is important to remember that the idea of singing or performing can bring up feelings of embarrassment or anxiety, so being alert to this in the room and supporting the child through this is essential.

Splat anger

This activity helps children and grownups explore the idea that angry feelings come and go.

What you need
Water balloons, an outdoor space and access to a tap, or a Buddha Board with a paintbrush and a cup of water.

Introducing this activity
There are a number of different ways to use this activity, meaning that you can choose an option that is likely to appeal to the child you are seeing and fit with the context you are working in.

The first option is to use water balloons, which works well with younger children and if you have an outdoor space. You can fill the balloons with the child, encouraging them to describe a time when they might get angry as they do so. You can fill the balloon to represent the size of their anger, making smaller balloons for smaller amounts of anger (such as annoyed or frustrated feelings) and bigger balloons for bigger amounts of anger (including furious or enraged feelings). It often helps if you fill a balloon for yourself first, naming something that makes you angry and choosing the appropriate size to fill the balloon to. Grownups might be encouraged to similarly fill some balloons as well. Filled balloons can be placed in a bucket ready for the next step in this activity.

The next step involves throwing the balloons at a wall or on the ground. You want a surface that will allow you to notice the wet patch that results and observe as it dries. You can then encourage the child to throw the balloons at the wall or on the ground. Once this is done you can notice the anger in the form of the water. You can notice with the child what it is like to see it there and how it feels to remember those situations you named. You might also notice that the smaller balloons left smaller splotches and the larger ones left larger splotches. Encourage the child to watch for any changes over time. For example, you might notice that the water marks initially took up six of the paving squares but that they are slowly fading.

A Buddha board is another way to do this activity in a more contained way and works well indoors if you don't have an outdoor space you can use. Sometimes older children prefer this option. Buddha boards come with a brush that can be dipped in water and used for drawing on a special board. You can encourage the child to splat blots of water to express their angry feelings. The board slowly dries and the drawing disappears, providing a similar experience to what a child might experience when watching water dry on a pavement. Buddha boards are readily available to buy online.

Considerations and adaptations
Grownups also benefit from remembering that anger comes and goes, so it can be helpful to engage them in this activity with the child, allowing them to watch some of their own anger fade too. Reflecting on how the child and grownup can remember this in moments of dysregulation can be helpful.

If you are working online, another option is to use Mindful Draw, which was created by Dr. Karen Fried (www.mindfuldraw.com). The brush style can be changed to blotter and the size can be altered, allowing the child to splat anger on the screen.

Getting in the tank

This activity is useful for helping children and grownups to explore their fight responses.

What you need
A toy army tank, preferably one that has a manhole marked on the top so that you can talk about how you get in the tank.

Introducing this activity
I usually begin this activity by suggesting we play with the tank and exploring whether the child has ever seen a tank in real life. Children have often seen a tank at a park or on television and have something to share about this. Asking questions that help them to notice how strong tanks are, how tanks are driven and how people get in and out of them is often helpful at this point. As the conversation progresses, we notice that the person driving the tank is really quite small in comparison to the tank and is just a regular person.

We then talk about how sometimes this can happen when we are angry: we quickly climb into a tank and start firing guns and cannons. Children might like to say some of the things that they might "shoot" at others when they are angry, enacting a battle with the tank as they do so. You can also encourage grownups to share about times when they find themselves climbing into the tank. I emphasize here that this reaction is understandable and is something that we can all find ourselves doing at times. We also talk about how we can notice that we might have climbed into the tank so that we can choose some more effective coping options.

Army tanks tend to wreak a lot of havoc and destruction and you may like to get curious about what it is like after a child has been in a tank, exploring the impact of what they have shot off in their moment of anger. Again, this is not about shaming the child, but is about providing some hope about how this could be different in future. For example, you might say something like "I know that you often feel bad later when you have shot all those words at Mom, and I think that we can work on you noticing when you are getting in the tank so this doesn't happen so often."

Considerations and adaptations
It can also be helpful to explore the responses of other family members, which can reduce the focus on the child and help them identify patterns. For example, grownups can also be encouraged to notice when they are feeling overwhelmed or unsafe and climb in their own tanks. Again, promoting an awareness can prompt grownups to make a different choice. They can also use this language with their child at home. For example, they might talk with a child about noticing that they might be climbing into the tank or reflecting on this after an angry outburst, depending on what is most appropriate.

Younger children will tend to engage in this activity in a more simplistic manner, and the conversations that they are able to have around this will be limited. This activity is likely to be most effective with them if used in the moment. For example, you might say something like "You've just started shooting all those words at Mom. It reminded me of my tank. Let's have a play with it and see if we can work out what is happening," before beginning to play with the tank together.

If you are working online, children might be engaged in this activity by looking at pictures of tanks online. Younger children may be less interested in this, though you may be able to have them show you their cars and you could then show them a tank of yours.

Tunnelling through the feeling

Children often feel uncomfortable about their anger and receive messages (some more overt than others) that the feeling is not ok. This activity is a useful way of demonstrating that anger is a feeling like any other and that we can allow ourselves to be curious about and learn from, rather than needing to avoid it or push it away.

What you need
A tunnel that is large enough for the child to safely and comfortably crawl through as well as some toy gems or gold pirate coins.

Introducing this activity
You can introduce this by asking the child if they would like to play with the tunnel and allow them to experiment with crawling through it or rolling a ball through it if they prefer. Suggest that you hide some treasure in the middle of the tunnel and ask how a child might be able to get the treasure. Typically, what happens as you do this is that children discover that they only get the treasure by crawling through the tunnel, collecting the treasure in the middle and continuing on the way out. You can wonder with the child about this experience and notice how they feel at different points. For example, some children might feel nervous as they begin to crawl into the tunnel and proud as they come out the other side with the treasure. They may feel curious or excited.

Once the child has experienced this, you can talk with the child and their grownups about how feelings are like this: there is often something important in a feeling that it can be helpful to find. Talk together about how, much like the experience of crawling through the tunnel, the only way to find it is to go through the feeling. You may also talk about the need to move slowly and look closely in order for the treasure or important meaning not to be lost.

Once the family are comfortable with this concept, you can talk about the important things we can learn from our angry feelings. For example, we might learn that there are worries or sad feelings hiding inside the angry feeling. We might also learn important information, such as understanding that a child feels overwhelmed by too many instructions, needs more warning when they need to move from one thing to another or needs more support at school.

Considerations and adaptations
Younger children are likely to enjoy crawling through the tunnel, though may need support to understand the idea of looking for what is important in their anger. For these children, you might like to use some messages written on small pieces of paper based on what you know about their anger. For example, messages like "I need a break" when placed in the middle of the tunnel can help children to reflect on what their anger might be communicating.

Families can be encouraged to continue talking about what is important in a child's anger at home. For example, they might be able to say "I can hear that it was important to you that your friend did not treat you that way"; they can then be encouraged to shape the child's behavioral response accordingly, perhaps saying something like "What might you be able to do next time?"

Angry balloon feelings

This activity is useful for helping children and grownups understand the cumulative nature of anger.

What you need
A balloon.

Introducing this activity
I introduce this activity by saying to the child and grownup that I've noticed that there are lots of small things that seem to annoy or frustrate them throughout the day. I draw on whatever language the family tends to use here and suggest that we take a balloon and blow that up as we talk so we can explore this more.

I then blow up the balloon asking about the annoyances and frustrations that the child has experienced in their day, blowing an amount of air into the balloon to symbolize this, checking with the child that I have blown in the correct amount of air. Holding the neck of the balloon to ensure that air does not escape as you check about the next annoyance is important so that you create a balloon that is gradually increasing in size with each annoyance that is blown into it. Younger children may need the support of grownups to share what is upsetting for them.

Encouraging the child to feel the outside of the balloon as you gradually fill it is often helpful. They might notice, for example, that it continues to feel soft early on though soon begins to feel a lot tighter. You can wonder with the child about whether there are similar changes in their body as the annoyances build up. I also encourage grownups to think of times where they have had a similar experience.

As the balloon becomes really big, you might notice that the child and/or grownup appear apprehensive, and checking in around this will often reveal some worry that the balloon is going to pop. This is often another good moment to pause and explore what might happen when there has been a build-up of annoyances.

Together, we begin to think about where there is anything that might release some of this tension, and I begin to slowly let out the air in response to calming activities or coping strategies described by the child and their grownup, again trying to let out an amount of air that symbolizes how helpful the child finds that approach. I continue to encourage the child to feel the balloon as it gradually goes down and again relate this to their experience. Grownups can also share what they have found helps release the tension for the child. At some point the child may identify a strategy they view as really helpful and say that I should let all the air out of the balloon, which can be fun to do by allowing it to fly around the room.

Considerations and adaptations
Most children enjoy this activity and are happy to name their annoyances. If they are less sure, though, you could have their grownup complete the activity first, sharing their own examples, or you

could demonstrate it yourself. Sometimes this activity has been particularly helpful for grownups who experience a build-up of stress over the day.

If families have a balloon available at home you could complete this activity online, asking the grownup to be responsible for blowing up the balloon.

Kindness binoculars

Kindness is not often an emotion that is evoked when dealing with anger. It is, however, often very helpful to view your own anger with kindness and to view others with kindness when you are angry. This activity helps children and grownups to view their anger through a lens of kindness.

What you need
Two cardboard rolls (e.g., paper towel rolls), craft glue, cellophane, a rubber band and markers.

Introducing this activity
I begin this activity by wondering about whether the child or their grownups have ever had the experience of using binoculars. I encourage them to share what this was like and reflect on how the binoculars changed how they saw things. I will generally begin by saying something about how I notice that sometimes it can be hard to see our anger with kindness. I will also notice that it can also be hard to be kind to others when we are angry. I then go on to suggest that we make some kindness binoculars that might help the child to see with kindness.

Make some simple binoculars by gluing together two cardboard rolls. A piece of colored cellophane can be secured across one end of the tubes with an elastic band and gives the child an experience of seeing things differently. I often encourage the child to decorate these binoculars, talking with them about what kindness means to them as they do so.

After making the binoculars, you can play with them, noticing how things look different when you look through them. Begin to play around with looking at situations using kindness. For example, if you are working with a child who likes to draw, you might like to look at a picture of the child getting angry, both with and without the kindness binoculars. Alternatively, for children who prefer imaginative play, you might like to act out situations using puppets or toys and watching these both with and without the kindness binoculars.

Children who communicate their needs or disappointment through their anger may be able to look at the situation and identify something like "I can see I was really upset then" or "Maybe I can tell Mom how much going to my friend's place meant to me." Through this, children can often see some of the feelings that underlie their anger, feel less ashamed about their feelings and begin to think of different ways in which they can communicate this.

Considerations and adaptations
Holding on to kindness while you are angry is also a helpful idea for those children who direct their anger toward others. Children might, for example, realize that they can be kind by thinking about those around them or remembering that sometimes these things happen.

Encouraging grownups to take a turn with the binoculars can be helpful too, and you may want to explore some of what they notice when they look at their own anger or their child's anger, depending on what is most relevant.

Reflecting on what it was like to use kindness binoculars is often helpful, getting curious about anything the child or family noticed. It is also worth talking to children about how they can use their kindness binoculars at home or at school. Thinking about when the binoculars might be most useful to the child and family is often helpful and can give you clues about how they could use the binoculars in their daily routine or where they might best sit in the house.

Sitting with all my feelings

This is a useful activity for helping children to notice their feelings, including anger, in the moment. It can also be useful for encouraging children to explore what anger might be communicating to them.

What you need

Two sets of small toys that depict different feelings—one set for you and one for the child. I have a set of small plastic figures, each of which has a different facial expression that corresponds to an easily recognized emotion. Another alternative is to use feeling cards, again having a set for you and one for the child.

Introducing this activity

It is helpful to explain to the child that you've noticed lots of feelings in the room and suggest that you each keep a set of figures with you, so that you can notice when these feelings come up. I would generally encourage children to choose a figure for happy, sad, worried and angry, though I would be guided by the language that they use around these feelings and would, of course, welcome the inclusion of other feelings. When grownups are also in the space, I encourage them to take a set of feelings too.

As we engage in the session I share when my feelings arise. For example, I might say "I noticed then that I felt really happy when you talked about winning the race at school" and hold up my happy figure, wondering aloud whether the child also had a happy feeling and encouraging them to hold it up if they did. Engaging in game play or in free play is often a good way to reflect on a range of emotions, encouraging the child to use their emotion figures when they notice feelings coming up in the room.

For children who need support to link what is happening with their body with their feelings, it is helpful to name this. For example, you might say something like "Hmm, I noticed your voice was a bit different then—is there a feeling that is coming up for you?" and encourage the child to look at their feelings. Children can also be encouraged to think about what their feeling might need or want. For example, I might say something like "Hi there, anger! It seems like you might want or need something. What is it?" and support the child to reflect on this. Often children might reflect that their anger is letting them know they need a break or want to play something different.

Considerations and adaptations

With younger children, it is important to keep the activity simpler. For example, you might focus just on helping a child identify the feelings. With an older child, however, you might be able to focus on identifying feelings and thinking about what they are communicating in the one session.

Having figures that clearly depict emotions reduces any requirement to remember which figures are which feelings, making this activity much easier. If you don't have sets of figures available, you could use cards, though keep in mind that figures are often more appealing, particularly for younger children. If you are working online, you could use a set of pictures that you have sent to the family ahead of time, keeping a set for yourself, so that you can both hold these up as the feelings arise.

You might like to encourage the child to take a photo of the feelings so they can remember to notice when these are coming up at home. Alternatively, if they have learnt something about their anger specifically, they may want to draw a picture to reflect this. For example, they might draw a picture of the angry feelings and write something like "Sometimes my anger wants me to let others know if I don't like something they are doing." If you have used cards for this activity, you may be able to send these home with the child.

It is also important to talk to grownups about how they might be able to notice the feelings that pop up, both for themselves and for their child.

How stretched are you today?

This activity is a useful way to help children and their grownups reflect on their window of tolerance. Having greater awareness of low levels of dysregulation can help grownups and children to draw on their coping strategies and adjust demands as needed.

What you need

A plastic Hoberman sphere (sometimes sold as an expandable ball) that can be collapsed or expanded.

Introducing this activity

I talk with the child about how some days we deal with lots of tricky or hard things and give some examples of this to show how these might build over time, expanding the ball to indicate an increased level of stress. I will often pause at this point and ask the child about stresses that build up over their day, making the sphere as big as they think it needs to be when I add each one, as seen in Figure 5.1.

We can also talk about how this works for the child's grownups, again using examples so that everyone understands the concept. For many families, this idea of stress building across the day or over time is an important one to understand, and you might choose to leave the activity here for a session, encouraging children and grownups to notice how stretched they are at a particular point in the day. You can talk about the sorts of things that stretch them and what it is like when they are stretched. It can be particularly helpful for grownups to be able to recognize when their children are in this state, so you might focus the conversation here if need be.

When children and grownups have had some time with this idea, you can begin talking about how hard it can be when you are already feeling stretched and other challenges come your way. Encourage the child and their grownups to think of examples of this as you hold the sphere in an almost fully stretched position and talk together about what might happen when further stresses are added. I will often encourage the child and family to hold the sphere at an almost fully stretched position and then stretch it out fully. You can explore what it is like to hold the sphere in that position by asking them to hold it there for a few minutes, noticing how they feel as they do so. Children and grownups will often notice the pain in their arms when doing this, and you can talk about the experience of being really stretched in this context. We can also play around with the idea of what might happen if there was one more stress that was added when the sphere is fully stretched. Children in this context will often talk about how it would break if they stretched it more and can relate this to times when they have had an angry outburst. This can facilitate a lot of helpful discussion around what children need in order to feel less stretched and can support the family to try some different approaches in this context.

Considerations and adaptations

Younger children can find it hard to relate their experiences to the ball so you might like to notice how stretched they are during the session, stretching the ball more in times of stress and decreasing it as they regulate to help them have a better sense of how this works. I will often use this approach if I am wanting to communicate this concept to the grownups, knowing that it will keep the child engaged and they will be more able to understand in this manner, whilst still allowing me to communicate with the grownups around this.

When children have engaged in this activity in sessions, they often enjoy communicating how stretched they are at the beginning of each session. They can often do so in online sessions too, instructing you to create the right size with the Hoberman sphere, when this has previously been introduced in a face-to-face session.

This activity is also very useful for grownups, and this might be your focus when using it. Helping a grownup to recognize when they are stretched and understand the way in which this influences their capacity to stay regulated in their interactions with their child can be very valuable. Recognizing when they need some time out or need to do something else to recharge can be invaluable.

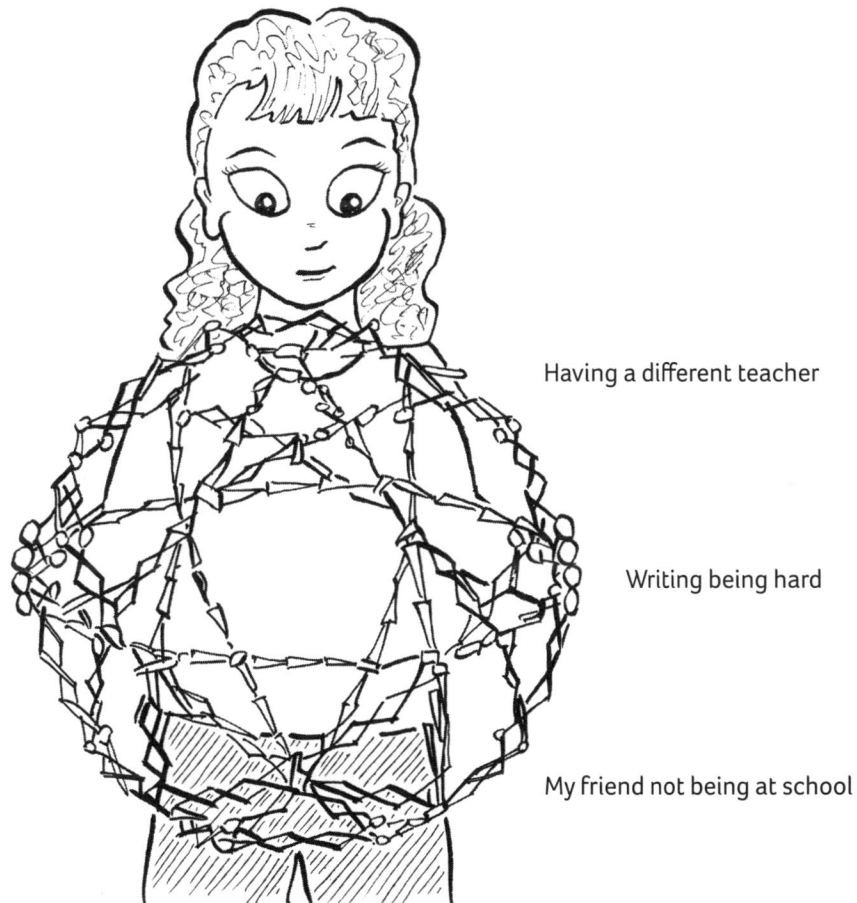

Having a different teacher

Writing being hard

My friend not being at school

FIGURE 5.1 USING THE EXPANDABLE BALL TO SHOW STRESSES

Magnifying feelings

Stressful situations can push us outside of our window of tolerance. This can include living through a pandemic, which was what prompted me to create this activity; however, children also face other longstanding stresses, including family conflict, social exclusion, illness and fatigue, all of which can leave them feeling stretched and make them more susceptible to becoming dysregulated in response to small triggers. This activity helps children and their grownups understand and explore this pattern.

What you need

A magnifying glass. You will also need some toys or other items to look at.

Introducing this activity

To introduce this activity, I take out my magnifying glass and allow the child to explore it. We choose some toys to look at using the magnifying glass and notice what happens. As we have the experience of seeing how much bigger things seem, I explain that the same thing happens when we are unwell/having a hard time at school/finding things challenging at home/whatever is relevant for the child. I encourage grownups to have a turn too and notice this pattern.

Older children might move at this point into discussing this, while younger children might benefit from exploring this more. We might, for example, write a trigger, such as being asked to unpack their bag, on a small slip of paper or choose something in the room that represents this, such as a figure to be their Mom asking this or a small bag. We notice how the magnifying glass makes this look so much bigger and that it feels quite overwhelming in that context. We will often label the magnifying glass as we play, saying things like "It's really quite small, but when I'm tired [holding the magnifying glass over the object as we say this] it seems like such a big thing." Grownups can also be encouraged to think about what magnifies their own angry feelings and can share their observations of what happens with the child in this space.

Considerations and adaptations

If you are working online you might like to use one of the online magnifying glasses to magnify parts of a screen that you are sharing or a picture the child has drawn.

Reflecting after this activity on how children and grownups can recognize when there might be something that is having a magnifying effect can be helpful. You can talk about how children can look after themselves when something is magnifying their feelings and how grownups can support them with this. For example, grownups might be able to notice when this is happening for the child and engage them in a regulating activity, reducing demands until the child is in a better space.

Unsafe animals

This activity is useful for exploring the idea that angry feelings occur when children feel unsafe.

What you need
Some animal figures or puppets.

Introducing this activity
I introduce this activity by suggesting that we play with some animals, taking out some animal figures or puppets. As we play, I begin to ask about what might happen when the animal feels unsafe. Children can often share some animal facts, and I encourage them to do so. When they are unsure I will often share some information. It's helpful to know how some animals typically respond here. As I am based in Australia, I often share that echidnas will curl themselves into a ball and may not move for some time when they feel unsafe. On the other hand, kangaroos might quickly hop away or might become aggressive when they feel unsafe.

The fight response, in which animals become mobilized in the context of feeling unsafe, is particularly helpful to explore with children who present with angry outbursts. Sharing that the fight response might not always be physical is important as some children who struggle with anger may engage primarily in verbal aggression.

Sharing some examples of responses and encouraging the child to think about times when they may have had a fight, flight or shutdown response can be helpful. Grownups can similarly reflect on their own responses. This is often a good opportunity to emphasize that a fight response occurs when children feel unsafe, not when they are making conscious choices.

Considerations and adaptations
Depending on the context, you may choose to do some reflection with the child and grownup together or do some with the grownup alone. Exploring why children might feel unsafe, despite appearing, objectively, to be safe, is often helpful in your discussions with grownups. This can also be a good chance to explore how grownups might be able to communicate to children that they are safe in this context.

Children often love animals and enjoy engaging in animal play, readily drawing connections between the play and their lives. Some grownups may, however, feel uncomfortable about being associated with animals, so do remain alert to this and adapt your approach as needed.

If you are working online, you may be able to engage older children in this activity while drawing animals or looking at pictures of them.

Understanding anger dice game

This activity supports children to understand more about their anger, using a simple game-like format. It is a useful way for children to explore and better understand their anger.

What you need

A foam dice, some paper, scissors and glue or some inexpensive dice and paper. You will also need some markers or pencils.

Introducing this activity

You can introduce this activity by suggesting that you make a game together so that you can learn more about anger. When using the foam dice you can suggest that you label each of the sides differently so that each roll of the dice helps you learn something different about anger. Together with the child, come up with prompts or questions that can be written on a piece of paper and glued onto a side of the dice. Work collaboratively and include the suggestions of the child and family; however, try to include what the anger feels like and how a child responds. For older children or those who have an awareness of their thoughts, it is also useful to include a prompt or questions that relates to the thoughts they have when they are angry. For example, your dice might include the following prompts:

1. *Look like* (so a child can show you what they look like when they are angry and you can build an awareness of their physiological symptoms)

2. *Say* (enabling a better understanding of their verbal behavior when angry)

3. *Do* (prompting the child to show or tell you how they behave)

4. *Feels like* (encouraging the child to put words to the feeling of anger)

5. *Thought* (supporting the child to identify the thought or thoughts associated with their anger)

6. *What helps* (helping the child to begin to build an awareness of regulation strategies)

If you are using regular dice you will need to create a playlist, similar to the one above. The playlist needs to include numbers 1–6 along with a prompt beside each so that when you roll the dice you can respond to the corresponding prompt.

The game is simple to play, with the child, any family members and yourself taking turns to roll and share about your own anger. Having a turn yourself allows you to engage in some teaching, helping the child to learn more about anger, and normalizes the experience of this emotion. The involvement of family members echoes this message and often allows for improved communication and greater empathy.

Considerations and adaptations

It is important to ensure that this is a positive experience for the child and is a good fit for them developmentally. You may need to support family members to share appropriate examples, either preparing them ahead of time or shaping their responses in the session. Keeping the child's developmental stage in mind when providing examples is also essential. For example, for a younger child, I will share simpler regulation strategies, such as asking someone for a hug; while for an older child, I might share something they can do more independently, like taking a breath and remembering they can handle this.

The particular prompts that you paste onto the dice will vary from child to child and should be influenced both by your awareness of the child and the stage of therapy. For example, a child who tends to get very stuck on their thoughts when they are angry may benefit from prompts that help them tune in to the emotional and physiological aspects of their experience. Similarly, a child who has a good awareness of their anger already may find it helpful to have more prompts around regulation on their dice.

If you are working online, you can roll a virtual dice and you can have the playlist handy while you roll.

Encouraging children to take the dice you have created or the list and a wooden or plastic dice home supports them to share this game with family members who have not been able to attend the session and helps them to generalize what they have learnt.

Different feeling parts

This activity helps children explore their feelings, encouraging them to see other feelings, such as disappointment, sadness or anxiety, that might go along with their anger. Increasing the complexity with which children understand their feelings and eliciting some conversation around this often helps them to better understand their anger. It also supports grownups to better understand their child's experience.

What you need

Blocks that connect, such as Lego or Duplo, or a blank jigsaw puzzle, the kind that can be purchased at craft stores.

Introducing this activity

How you introduce this activity will depend on where you are at with the child in therapy. For example, you might say that you've heard a lot about their angry feelings and are keen to explore some of their other feelings and suggest that you use some blocks to do so. Alternatively, you might introduce this while you are playing with blocks by saying something like "All of these pieces are reminding me of how sometimes different parts of me feel differently" and offering an example of this.

Offering an example is a good way to start. Finding something that the child can relate to is important. You could talk, for example, about being excited about catching up with a friend only to have your friend cancel. You can then go on to talk about how part of you felt disappointed, placing another block on the table as you do so, and reflecting on how much you had been looking forward to catching up. Then you might talk about how you also felt a bit angry, perhaps noting that your friend does sometimes cancel with little notice, fitting another block on top of the other to represent the angry feeling. You could then talk about feeling a bit worried as you take another block and fit it with the others, commenting that you sometimes worry about whether they really do care about you. If you are using a jigsaw puzzle you can have the child draw or write a feeling on each piece as they complete the puzzle.

The way in which you talk about each feeling should be varied according to the child's needs. For example, it is often helpful to comment on thoughts for children who are older; while if you have a child who is learning to recognize feelings in their body, you might describe these.

When the child has understood the concept, encourage them to think about the different feelings they might have experienced. It can be useful to talk about past situations and explore how all the different parts of them felt. Sometimes children will find it easier to explore hypothetical situations and to reflect on how the different parts of them might feel in that situation. Whichever way you approach this, the emphasis needs to be on helping a child to develop a more complex understanding of their anger, identifying the feelings that might underlie or be associated with this. Grownups can be encouraged to share examples of their own or to wonder about other feelings the child might have had in a specific situation.

Considerations and adaptations

If you are working online, you might need to check that the family has some blocks at home and ask that they have them ready ahead of the session.

Developmentally, older children are more able to understand mixed feelings and will be able to draw upon this when completing this activity. Some will, however, be overwhelmed by their anger, so eliciting some of the other feelings they experience is particularly helpful. Younger children are likely to need greater support with this activity, and your focus might need to be on helping their grownups to think about what the child might be feeling in addition to their anger.

Talking about the different parts of us and how they are feeling is really useful language to carry throughout your work with children and families. You can, for example, wonder about other parts of the child's experience when grownups describe an angry outburst. In the room with a child you might get curious about feelings they present, wondering how the other parts of them felt. You can also encourage the family to consider how they can notice the other feeling parts at home.

Baby babushka feelings

Anger is typically a secondary emotion, and identifying the emotions underneath can help children connect with their feelings and communicate them with others. This activity helps children to connect with these feelings in a playful way.

Babushka dolls are often used in therapy, particularly in Gestalt therapy (e.g., Day and Day 2012), and having a set can be particularly helpful. This particular activity, however, was inspired by Karen Treisman (2017), who utilized these dolls to help children think about the different feelings that were under their defensive response or anger.

What you need

Some babushka dolls to play with or the template that follows and markers or pencils.

Introducing this activity

You can introduce this activity by asking if the child has ever seen a babushka doll and wondering if they would like to see one. Show the child a set of babushka dolls, talking as you play about how the dolls hide within each other. You can then explain that feelings sometimes hide under anger and begin to explore this idea. You may like to use stickers to draw different feelings and stick these on the dolls, drawing an angry feeling for the outside and helping the child to identify a feeling that might be underneath their anger and sticking that feeling on the doll inside. There are also plain wooden sets available that children can decorate. Another option is to use the template provided here. The child can decorate the card, illustrating the inside to show the feeling underneath their anger. If you are working online and can share the template ahead of time and the family can complete this activity in their session with you.

For some children, you might like to give an example of a time when you felt angry and describe the feeling underneath prior to asking them about a time in which they felt angry. For others, it might be preferable to refer to a recent situation in which they were angry and explore this.

It is helpful to encourage some play with the babushka dolls. Again, this should be targeted to what you think the child most needs. For example, children who need to develop compassion for themselves might benefit from taking the role of the underneath doll in play; while children who need support to communicate their feelings to others might experiment doing so with each of the dolls and explore whether it is easier to communicate their feelings with others when they are angry or disappointed. Similarly, you might use this activity if one of your goals is around developing the grownups' awareness of the child's experience, helping them to focus on the feeling underneath the child's anger as you complete this activity together. Grownups can also benefit from connecting with the feelings underneath their anger and may find it helpful to complete their own babushka or at least reflect on the feelings underneath their anger.

Considerations and adaptations

If you are working online you may be able to send a copy of the template to the family ahead of time or ask if they have babushka dolls at home that could be used in the session.

When reflecting, it is also helpful to encourage the child and family to think about how they can better connect with the feelings underneath their anger. You might, for example, talk with grownups about how they can connect with the feelings underneath, using strategies such as hugging their child or breathing with them when they are dysregulated. Children may also be able to share more of their underlying feelings with their grownups, providing their grownups with a much better sense of their triggers.

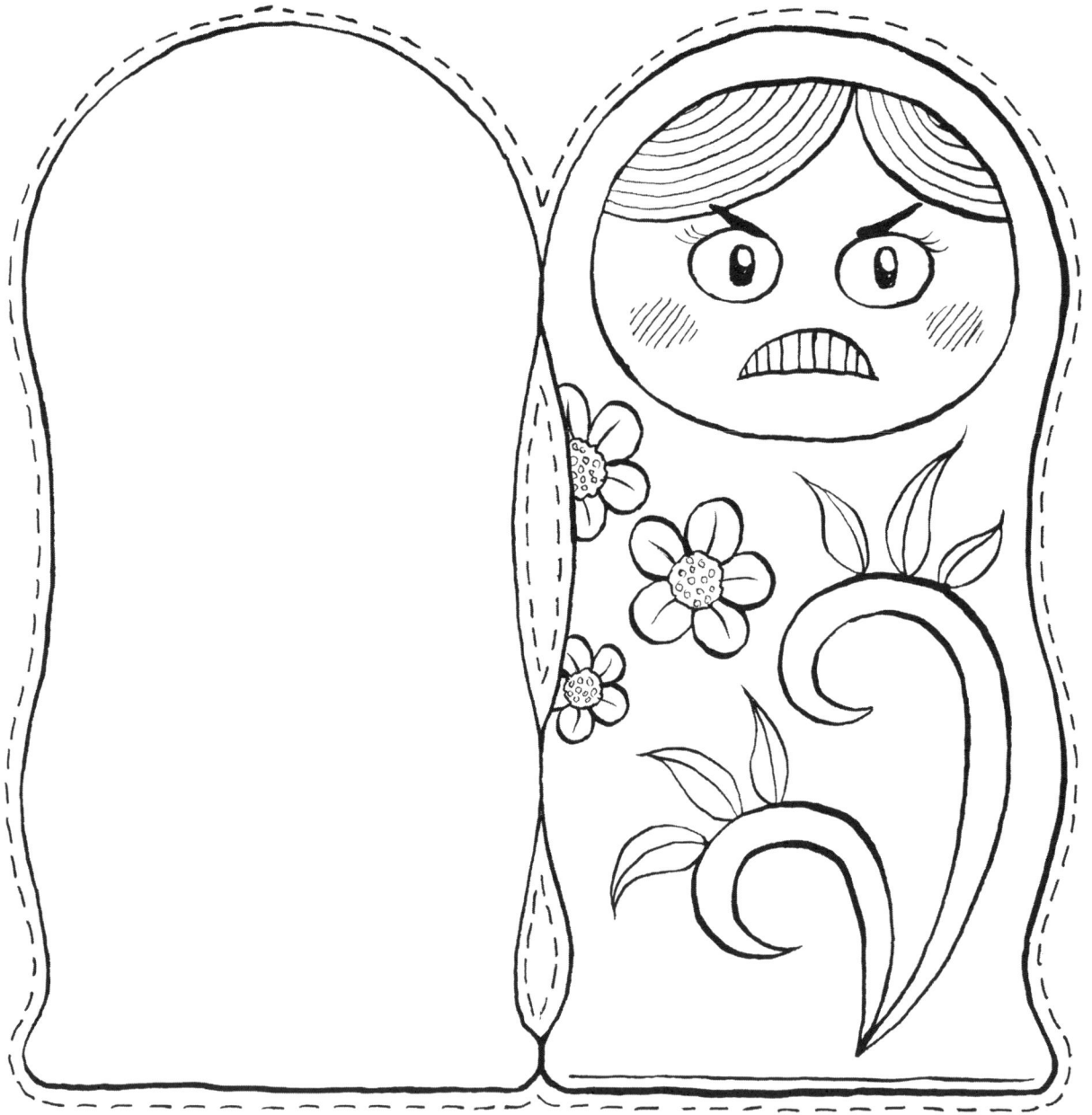

Seeing the other feelings in my anger

This activity helps children and their families to understand the other feelings that may be hiding underneath their anger. Understanding that anger is a secondary emotion is often helpful for children and their families and can create greater empathy and opportunities for communication.

What you need
Some paper and color change markers. If you don't have color change you can use regular markers.

Introducing this activity
You can introduce this activity by noticing that you have been talking a lot about anger and are wondering if you can explore this further. Encourage the child to write the word ANGER in big block or bubble letters so that you can talk about this further. Younger children may want help to do this, while others may prefer you to write the letters. *Anger* is the word I've chosen in writing up this activity, however in practice it is helpful to use whatever word the family tends to use, whether this be *Mad*, *Rage* or *Meltdown*.

If you have color change markers, allow the child to color the letters of the word ANGER with the colored markers. As they are doing so, wonder together about whether there may be other feelings underneath the anger or hiding inside of it and suggest that you use the white color change marker to uncover these. Family members can be engaged in this discussion too. It is often helpful to consider some past examples of anger and get curious about whether there were some other feelings, such as worry or sadness, that were underneath the anger on those occasions. Sharing some examples of when anger has been a secondary emotion for you is often useful in facilitating the conversation, and family members may be encouraged to do similarly. Sharing your observations of times when the child has been angry and your guesses about the other feelings under this is often helpful.

As the child and family members identify emotions, you can use the white marker to write these feeling words within the block or bubble writing, as in Figure 5.2. The white marker changes the color of the other markers. For example, it might turn purple to pink, allowing you to notice how these feeling words magically appear as though they were previously hidden. Some children may like to draw feeling faces rather than write the words.

Encouraging family members to wonder about the other feelings that might be in a child's anger and creating a space to talk and connect around these is often helpful.

Considerations and adaptations
If you don't have color change markers available you can write the feeling words within the bubble or block writing. This can also be done on a shared whiteboard if you are working online.

When completing this activity, I talk often with the family about anger more generally, drawing the hidden feelings in as we discuss a range of different examples and explore broadly some of the feelings that might be under their child's anger. For some grownups, however, it is more helpful to explore one situation at a time, listing the feelings that may have been hidden in their child's anger on that occasion prior to considering another example.

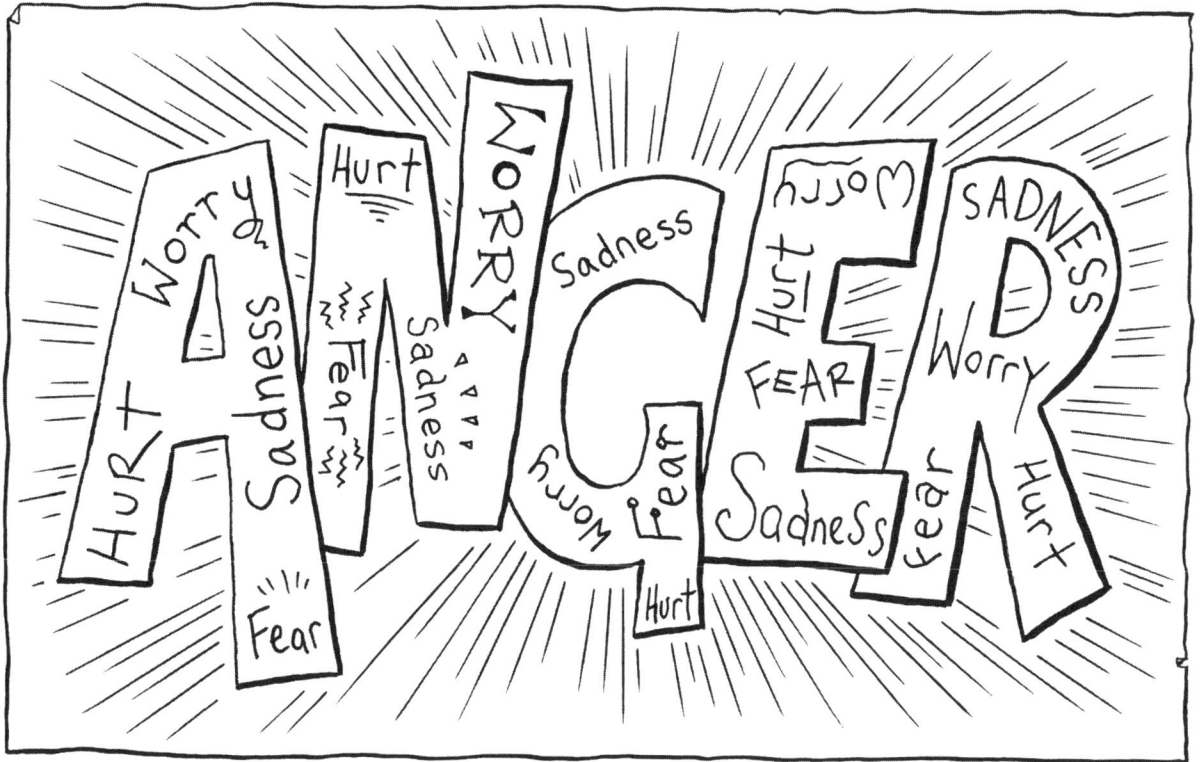

FIGURE 5.2 USING COLOR CHANGE MARKERS TO SEE THE FEELINGS IN MY ANGER

Clouds of anger

This is a useful activity for helping children and families to explore how stress can build up over time, eventually raining down as anger. It is helpful for children who tend to have cumulative stresses which build until the time they are quite dysregulated and respond by becoming very angry in response to a small trigger.

What you need
Paper and some markers or pencils.

Introducing this activity
You can introduce this activity using some paper and markers or pencils, suggesting that you draw as you talk. Encourage the child to draw some pictures of the weather with you. You can chat about the weather, getting curious about what weather the child likes best and how they feel about the rain. If the child has not spontaneously drawn any rain clouds encourage them to do so or draw one yourself. You can also ask about whether the child knows how clouds work. A simplistic explanation is that clouds are made of water droplets and when these become too heavy they rain down to earth. Explain to the child that sometimes we experience lots of little sadnesses, annoyances and frustrations, and that they can become heavier and heavier until finally they rain down. List some of the experiences you have that sometimes add to your own anger and encourage the child's grownups to reflect appropriately on their own if they are in the session.

You can also talk about how it feels when you are like a really heavy rain cloud and are ready to rain or even storm, encouraging the child to tune in to what this feels like in their body. Encouraging grownups to reflect on what they notice when the child is experiencing a build-up of frustrations that are about to rain down can also be helpful. Grownups can also share about their own experience of this.

These discussions help the family to better understand what a child finds stressful, to notice early warning signs and reflect on strategies they can use to support the child. It also encourages children to reflect on this for themselves.

Considerations and adaptations
Developmentally, older children will be able to engage in more conversation around this, while younger children will likely talk less, focusing more on drawing their clouds. Regardless, the activity provides a useful way to talk about anger, one which often works better for children and families, providing a playful distance and enabling greater space for reflection.

If you are working online, you may like to draw on an online whiteboard or look at pictures of different weather conditions as you talk.

The washing machine

This activity is useful for children who tend to ruminate on angry, sad or worried thoughts. Rumination often increases agitation and can result in angry outbursts. It is therefore helpful for children and grownups to be aware of this pattern and how they might be able to shift it. Smith (2022) uses the metaphor of a washing machine to describe rumination, and I have expanded on this here, adapting it to make it playful and engaging for children.

What you need
Paper, or the template on the next page, and markers or pencils.

Introducing this activity
I introduce this activity by noticing that a child seems to be going round and round with their thoughts. Ask about whether they have a washing machine at home and whether they have ever noticed how the clothes do this. Most children have observed their grownups doing the laundry and many have seen the washing moving through the window at the front of the washing machine. Children may like to draw a picture to show you what their washing machine looks like or color in the template. I often encourage children to make the round and round motion with their bodies. Encouraging the child to name some of the thoughts that are going round and round for them, drawing a picture to represent these or writing these inside the machine can be helpful.

I then link this motion with the experience of having angry, sad or worried thoughts that go round and round. Encouraging the child to share how they feel when this happens, share about your own experience of this process, and invite grownups to share about when this happens to them. It is often useful at this stage for therapists to share gently some of what they notice about the child when this happens.

Once children are familiar with this concept, it is helpful to talk together about what the washing machine does when it is done with the round and round washing cycle. I explain that the washing machine switches at this point and drains and spins. Demonstrating these actions with your body is often helpful. For example, we might enact the draining action by dropping our shoulders and arms and taking a deep breath out. This often leads to a helpful conversation about stopping and engaging in a different action.

Considerations and adaptations
It is helpful to notice the washing machine pattern as it occurs in the room and continue this language through your work with the child and family. Talking about those times when you are 'in the washing machine' is a playful way to notice this and children often respond well to this. Creating space for noticing and working through this, suggesting they might like to try a different action, is useful and supports the child and family to generalize these skills. The family can also be encouraged to use this language at home, noticing when someone in the family is in the washing machine and thinking about a course of action that might help.

If you are working online, you might invite a child and grownup to show you their washing machine, or you can share the washing machine template ahead of time.

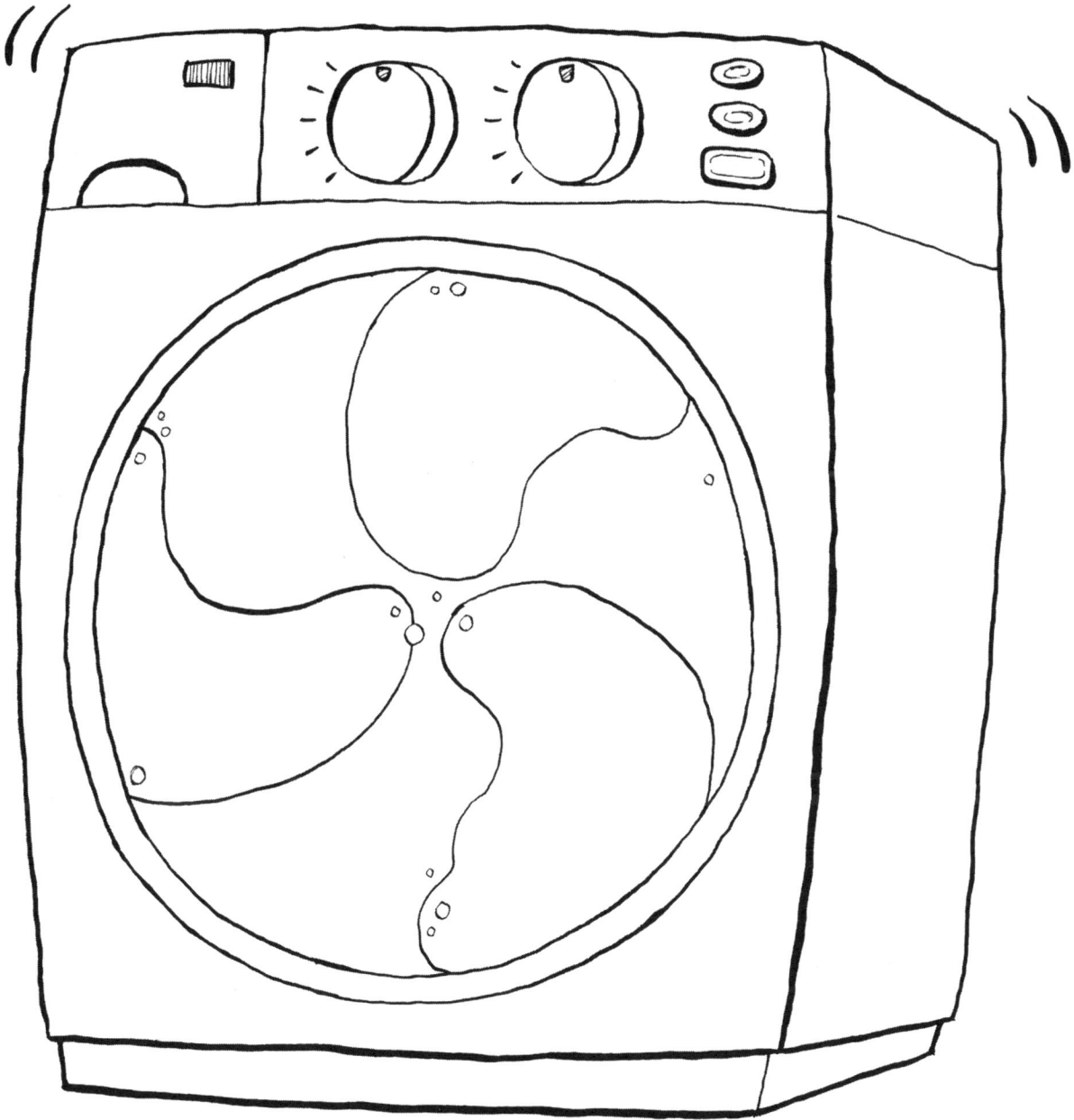

Spinning anger

Children (and grownups) lack the ability to see situations clearly when they are really angry, which often makes it difficult for them to make good choices. This activity makes use of a simple science experiment, referred to as Newton's disc, to help them understand why it can be helpful to slow down and regulate when they are angry.

What you need

The template on the next page printed on light cardboard, some scissors, markers or pencils, and a paper drinking straw.

Introducing this activity

You can introduce this activity by saying that you have noticed that when people get angry it can be hard to think or see a situation clearly. Suggest that together you make something that spins quickly to explore this idea. Have the child color each of the sections in a single color. The experiment needs all the colors of the rainbow: red, orange, yellow, green, blue, indigo and violet, as marked in the example on the template.

Once the card has been colored, cut it out, making a hole in the center, as shown on the wheel. Insert a paper drinking straw through the middle at the marked point. Spin the stick fast by rubbing it between your hands or fingers and notice the colors. When spun quickly, the color of the wheel appears to be a white or grey with the colors disappearing.[2]

As you play with the spinning disc with the child and family, you can notice how the colors disappear and that they become hard to see. It is helpful to reflect on other times when it is difficult to see things clearly and encourage the family to think about how they see situations when they are angry or dysregulated. Grownups can be asked to provide examples too if they are involved in the session.

Considerations and adaptations

In reflecting on this activity, it can be helpful to think about how the child and their grownups can remember that being really dysregulated makes it difficult to see and think clearly. This can prompt some discussion around pausing when we are angry so that we can think about what the feeling is telling us and make a choice around how we want to respond. You can encourage some reflection around how we can notice when we are spinning in anger and the ways in which we can slow down, such as pausing and breathing. Practicing this in the session as the disc spins can be helpful.

---

2   For information about the science behind this as well as instructions on how to create a disc, go to: www.fizzicseducation.com.au/150-science-experiments/light-sound-experiments/newton-colour-wheel

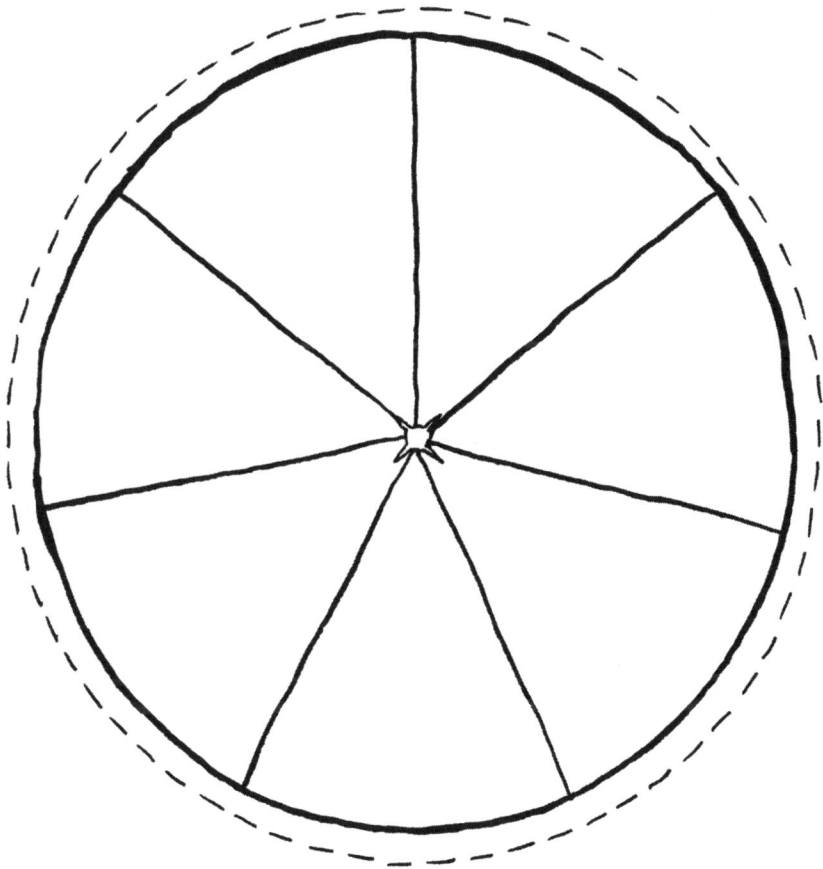

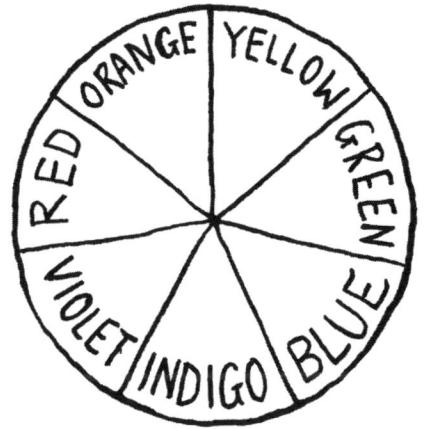

See it differently

This activity helps children and families to see their child's anger differently. It is particularly useful for uncovering positives in a child's anger or thinking about what other emotions might be contained within this.

What you need
A kaleidoscope.

Introducing this activity
I typically introduce this idea as the child or family talks about the anger, wondering whether there might be other ways to see what is happening. You can ask if the child and family have ever seen a kaleidoscope and suggest that they might like to see how it works or have a play with it. Notice the family's responses and discover together that, although there are no new shapes in the kaleidoscope, as you twist it the kaleidoscope reveals very different patterns.

You can then link this experience with how the child's anger is perceived. I will do this by sharing something that is relevant to the child's behavior and offering another way to view this. For example, I might share that I've noticed that the child tends to become angry in the lead-up to social events and wonder if they might be anxious about these, that I'm wondering if their anger might be their way of setting some boundaries with their peers, or that I can see that they've needed to protect themselves in the past and that their anger has allowed them to do so, depending on what is most relevant. Noticing that the behavior is not different, rather it is the lens you are looking through, reassures the family that you are seeing what they see, despite perhaps viewing it in a different way. It also opens up the possibility for the family to view the behavior differently. You may, for example, wonder with a family who are very focused on a child's behavior about whether they could see the behavior through an emotional lens and encourage them to get curious about how their child might be feeling. This may help them to appreciate how challenging these moments are for the child or support them to understand the anxiety or sadness that might be within the anger.

Considerations and adaptations
Younger children might struggle to engage in this conversation and it might be more developmentally appropriate to direct this at the grownups. Most will, however, enjoy playing with the kaleidoscope and the experience of seeing it change as they turn it, so it may still be appropriate to have them in the room. It can also help older children to see other feelings within their anger or recognize what their anger might be communicating to others. For example, you could say something like "It's a bit like when you stormed out of class. I can look at that as you doing the wrong thing and not following the teacher's rules, but I can also look at it another way and see that you really needed a break."

When reflecting on this activity, it is helpful to encourage the family to be curious about what it is like to see the behavior differently. Wondering about different ways of seeing it is often useful for both the child and the grownups.

Who's that knocking?

This is a useful activity for helping children to get curious about their anger and explore what this feeling might be telling them. It is particularly useful for children who are reluctant to explore their anger, providing them with some distance using a narrative approach and allowing them to titrate their experience by gradually opening the door a little more. It was inspired by Laura Rubenstein's delightful picture book *Visiting Feelings* (2013).

What you need
Paper and markers or pencils, clay or puppets.

Introducing this activity
I introduce this activity by saying to children that you can hear there is some anger there and wondering if we could think about this as a visitor who is knocking at the door. You can then begin to wonder about this visitor. For example, you might ask how that feeling would knock on the door and try some different sorts of knocks until you find the right one.

You can also get curious about the following points:

- What size would the anger be—would it fill the doorway or easily come through?

- What form might the anger take—is there a person, character or animal that it might look like?

- What sort of voice might the anger use—what sort of words might it use, would it be a louder voice or a softer one?

You can encourage the child to draw a picture of anger or mold it with some clay. Alternatively, the child may prefer to find a puppet or figure in the room to symbolize it. Looking at the picture or pretending the character is knocking on the door can be helpful and is a good opportunity to pause and reflect on any feelings or thoughts that come up for the child as anger knocks on the door.

Reflecting on how the child feels about opening the door is helpful at this point. Do they feel ok to open it and learn more about why anger is there? Or does letting anger in feel too overwhelming and would they prefer to look through the intercom or through the peephole? Perhaps they just want to open the door a little and look out while keeping the chain on. Exploring this helps give you a sense of how comfortable the child is with their anger. It allows you to suggest options such as just glancing quickly at anger through the window as a way of encouraging them to briefly engage with, and get curious about, anger.

Encouraging children to at least open the door a tiny crack can bring them back to the purpose or function of their anger. Asking questions like "Why is anger knocking on the door?", "What might anger want you to know?", "Is there anything anger needs?" and "What might anger want you to do or say?" can prompt some useful discussion and reflection around this.

Considerations and adaptations

This activity often works best with older children, given the language and imagination required. More generally however, the idea of anger being a visitor is a useful one and can be adapted for younger children. For example, you might emphasize the role of feelings telling us something important, coming back to this idea and integrating this throughout your sessions with a younger child.

Drawing on a shared whiteboard is a useful way to approach this activity if you are working online.

Getting comfortable with uncomfortable feelings and thoughts

This activity acknowledges when children feel uncomfortable sharing about angry feelings or thoughts and provides children with an opportunity to understand and relate to these feelings and thoughts in a different way. It is particularly helpful for children who avoid talking about their uncomfortable angry feelings.

What you need
Calming options, such as cushions, a blanket, soft toys and sensory items.

Introducing this activity
This activity is most useful when uncomfortable angry feelings and thoughts arise in the session. When this occurs, you can say something like "It looks like this is really hard to talk about/think about/ draw. I wonder if there is anything we can do to make this easier. Let's all try to get as comfortable as we can while we talk about/think about/draw this uncomfortable stuff."

I then encourage the child to think about what might make them a bit more comfortable. I also explain that their grownups and I will get comfortable in preparation for talking about the uncomfortable angry thoughts. For example, they may want to move closer to their grownups, hold their hand, have their back rubbed or have a cuddle. They may want to choose a cushion or a soft toy to hold while they talk or may want something to fidget with. Having items such as cushions, soft toys and sensory toys is likely to be very helpful; however, it is also useful to reflect on internal resources too. For example, children might like to take some deep breaths or move their bodies as they talk. I encourage the grownups to think about what they need to do in getting ready to talk and model strategies as I prepare myself for talking about the uncomfortable feelings and thoughts too.

Once the child is comfortable, you can begin to lean in to the uncomfortable feelings or talk about the uncomfortable thoughts more. As you do so, it is important to carefully notice how the child is responding so that you can keep them attuned to their body and help them find ways to regulate. For example, you might say something like "I think that sitting on Dad's lap has really helped—you've been able to talk more about how disappointed and angry that makes you." Similarly, if a child has been regulated and then begins to become dysregulated again you might say something like "That cushion was making it easier. You told me a bit about what happened at school, but now your voice is getting louder and you're talking a lot faster. Do you think that we need to do something else to help us while we talk about this?"

What often happens as we talk about the uncomfortable angry feelings is that they become easier to talk about. Noticing this pattern is worthwhile and can help to reduce some of the feelings that children have around anger.

Considerations and adaptations

It is important that we never pressure children to say more than they want to. Giving them the choice of how much they share or don't share creates safety within the therapeutic relationship. This activity is not about pressuring children to talk about feelings, thoughts or experiences they are not ready to share; rather it is about helping to make it a bit easier for them to share what they choose to.

This activity requires very little modification for online use. Indeed, helping a child to get comfortable at home has the distinct advantage of allowing you to better understand the home setting and supports them to generalize from the session to their day-to-day life. Having a grownup available to support the regulation can also be very helpful.

CHAPTER 6

RESPONDING TO ANGER IN THE ROOM AND SUPPORTING GROWNUPS TO RESPOND

Moments of dysregulation are to be expected in therapy sessions when working with emotional dysregulation. In this chapter I share some considerations around responding to anger in sessions and the role of limit-setting. A model for helping grownups to regulate their children is also included.

Responding to anger in sessions

MAYA

Maya came into the clinic room without greeting me. She began moving about in an agitated way, going from one activity to another and handling the toys roughly. I remembered that she was said to present this way when she was angry and wondered out loud about this. As her mother began telling me about what had happened that morning, Maya charged at her and began hitting her. Her mother began to tell her off as I took a breath and suggested we find something to calm Maya's body, passing her some cushions as I did so. As she began to bang the cushions on the couch, Maya began to calm, and I shared what I noticed about her body movements and breathing to help both Maya and her mother recognize these signs. Her mother began to describe what had made Maya angry. Reflecting that I had noticed that Maya found it difficult to talk about her feelings, I suggested that we create a safe space for Maya so that we could look after her as her mother shared what had happened. We built a small cubby on the couch using the cushions for Maya to hide in and found a way that her mother could reach in and rub her back as we talked about what had happened.

Children may become angry in therapy sessions for a number of reasons. Indeed, it is unsurprising that if we are working with children who are learning to regulate their emotions we are likely to see their anger arise at times. Sometimes the triggers for a child's anger occur during a therapy session. For example, a child who struggles with things not being clear and there being some uncertainty may find it challenging when a therapist asks an open-ended question about their feelings and may respond by becoming anxious and angry.

Sometimes we have an awareness of a child's triggers ahead of time; at other times these become apparent in the session. Furthermore, even when we are aware of a child's triggers it is not always possible to avoid these in sessions. For example, when a child struggles with transitions and often becomes dysregulated in this context, we can provide lots of warning and scaffolding though cannot eliminate transitions entirely. Each session contains at least two potential triggers for these children: namely, coming into the room and leaving the room. Taking the time to work through triggers and support the child to regulate through this is often helpful.

Given the nature of child work, there are likely to be times, as in the example above, where we are faced with family members expressing anger toward each other. As therapists, we can make observations that help the child and family to better understand what is happening. For example, you might notice that the grownup seems to be offering lots of logical arguments at a time when the child is dysregulated and not able to engage in this sort of conversation. You may be able to gently suggest some calming time or offer the child a soft toy or cushion during the session, encouraging the grownup to wait before speaking further. Reflecting once you've been able to work through this and being curious about whether there is a similar pattern at home is often helpful and enables you to work with the child and family about how they can best manage dysregulation at home.

As in the above example, observing anger in sessions also gives us a better understanding of what is happening in families and can help us understand what a child and family most need. By the time children come to therapy, patterns of responding to the anger have often become deeply ingrained, and grownups may struggle to reflect on what occurs in these moments and identify what might need to change, so being able to observe patterns is incredibly helpful.

Even when grownups have been able to provide a clear description of their interactions with their child when they are angry, having this happen in the session provides an opportunity for responding differently. Grownups sometimes also need scaffolding, and having a therapist who can slow down the interaction and model some regulation strategies can be powerful. Like children, grownups too have often developed automatic ways of responding to their child's anger. Exploring alternatives and practicing these in sessions gradually builds their capacity to respond in a more useful manner.

Far more important than the words we say is what we do in therapy. Ensuring that our actions mirror our words helps to create safety and predictability for children and families. It adds depth to our work and allows us to be authentic. Sometimes, without intending to do so, we say one thing only to demonstrate another. As in the example provided in Chapter 1, where Lucy talked about everyone getting angry and then proceeded to only focus on the child's anger, inconsistencies often sit uncomfortably for children and families. Ensuring that you embody what you say helps to create safety for our clients, and it is useful to reflect on how you do this in your practice. As in the example of Lucy, providing space to explore each family member's anger and provide appropriate examples of your own is a good way of reinforcing the idea that everybody experiences anger. Similarly, pausing and getting curious about what a child or grownup's anger might be communicating when it arises in a session emphasizes the idea that anger is important and that we can be curious about it.

Setting limits in therapy and helping grownups to do so

"Wait, we need a rule," screams one of the 10-year-old girls as they careen around the house in what must be the noisiest sleepover I have hosted. Clearly, something in the frenzied chase-each-other-in-the-dark game they are playing is not working and there needs to be some further negotiation. I marvel at the wisdom of this simple comment: the implicit understanding that boundaries and limits need to be set as needed. I too have set a limit, flagging for the girls that in around an hour they'll need to do something quieter in their beds, knowing that there is only so much excited screaming and hurtling through the house all of us can manage.

SIOBHAN

Siobhan was clearly dysregulated when she entered the clinic room. She moved in an agitated manner around the room and began throwing toys around. I noticed her need to throw and provided her with some soft balls. She threw them hard and one nearly hit the light, which prompted me to encourage her to find a space in which she could safely throw the balls. Siobhan threw the balls hard at the blanket her aunt and I held up between us, doing so for a few minutes before she gently rubbed the blanket against her face. I noticed that she liked the feel and let Siobhan know that she could wrap herself in it if she would like to do so. She draped it over her head and shoulders like a hooded cape and settled into playing with some other toys.

Limits are important. Grownups who have limits help ensure that children are safe and that their needs are met. Goodyear Brown (2021) refers to this as playing the role of *safe boss*, with grownups needing to be both a secure base and a safe haven for their children, as described in the Circle of Security model (Hoffman *et al.* 2017). One of the important functions of being a safe boss is setting clear limits when needed (Goodyear Brown 2021). Landreth (2023) makes the point that limits are not needed until they are, which is apparent in the two scenarios described above. Dion (2018) also points out that we need to set a limit when not doing so would push us outside of our window of tolerance and lead to us being dysregulated. The girl I described in the sleepover above was becoming dysregulated by the chaotic nature of the play and responded by setting a limit. Similarly, mindful of where I was at, I also set a limit. Seen in this context, limits create safety by preventing dysregulation.

When talking with grownups about where the limits need to be, therefore, my primary consideration is around safety. In addition to physical safety, however, limits also provide emotional and relational safety. I encourage grownups who are dysregulated by their child's behavior to notice this and to set a limit, noting their child's need and redirecting it so that they are able to remain present for their child. In response to the question about where a limit needs to be, my answer is often around where the limit needs to be in order for both the child and the grownup to remain safe and regulated. This is not to say that I don't at times explore the limits a grownup has set and encourage greater flexibility. For example, I might talk about the role of chaotic or noisy play with a grownup who quickly imposes limits on this. My emphasis is on helping the grownup to tune in to their responses and set limits where they need to before gradually trying to widen their window of tolerance.

Having limits is important, but the way in which limits are set is also important. Holding the child's needs in mind when setting limits often helps us to remain attuned whilst keeping them safe. This is about noticing what the child needs and helping them find a safe way to have these needs met. Landreth (2023) proposes that in setting limits we need to acknowledge the child's feelings, wishes and wants, communicate the limit and target acceptable alternatives. Dion (2018) has suggested using the language of "finding another way" when a child needs to be redirected, which often works well in the therapy space. As in the example of Siobhan, this allows us to acknowledge a child's need whilst creating boundaries as needed.

When children are dysregulated, limit-setting needs to occur alongside acknowledging their needs and empathizing with their feelings. The HOLDS model presented below provides a framework for helping grownups to regulate their child.

Helping grownups to regulate their children using HOLDS

The HOLDS acronym was developed through my work with grownups. It provides a broad framework that has key steps, whilst allowing grownups to personalize each of these elements, finding what works for themselves and their child. The word *hold* evokes a helpful image too, positioning the grownup as bigger, stronger and wiser and able to support the child through the big emotions they are experiencing. This is consistent with the Circle of Security model, which talks about holding as keeping the child safe and protected whilst they experience overwhelmingly big feelings (Hoffman *et al.* 2017). HOLDS stands for:

- **H**aving a moment to connect with your own feelings and look after yourself.

- **O**rganizing the child's feelings, as well as the situation.

- **L**ooking for the feelings underneath.

- **D**oing the things that are regulating.

- **S**peaking after the child and grownup are regulated.

It is important to note that holding describes the emotional experience, rather than the physical one in this context, though providing physical comfort may indeed be nurturing for some children and may be something that children benefit from in this context. It is also important that grownups understand that this model is not for those times when there are immediate safety risks. If a child is about to run across a busy road in a moment of anger, it is essential that we stop them from doing so straight away, rather than attempt to co-regulate them through this situation.

The elements of the HOLDS model are discussed below, along with some considerations for using it. A handout for grownups describing this approach is also included.

H is for Having a moment to connect with your own feelings and look after yourself

It's natural for grownups to feel heightened when their child is angry. Behavioral and physiological synchronicity is often demonstrated between infants and parents in research studies and, while further research is needed (Bell 2020), this finding is consistent with what we often see in therapy. Grownups generally become activated when their child is angry and dysregulated, and calm as their child calms. In some ways this pattern of increased activation in response to children being dysregulated is helpful. It provides useful information about the child's experience and prepares the grownup to support the child. Reflecting on the tendency for grownups to catch their child's anger is often worthwhile, and learning why this might be important can be a valuable reframe for some grownups. Using some of the activities in Chapter 2 to explore this, such as *The shape of my anger* or *My anger is…*, can be helpful. The *Yawn game*, in which families use yawns to explore the way in which feelings catch in families (Zandt and Barrett 2017), is also particularly useful here.

Equally, it is important to acknowledge that grownups who become dysregulated in response to their child's anger find it harder to regulate their child. Given that grownups tend to calm as children calm, promoting the idea that grownups need to be calm in order to regulate children is unhelpful. Instead I encourage them to connect to their own feelings and those of their child so that they can be regulated enough to be able to manage this thoughtfully. Grownups who take a moment to connect with how they are feeling and take a deep breath in the face of their child's anger are unlikely to be calm; they are, however, likely to be in a space where they can connect with their own and their child's feelings, engage with their child in a supportive manner, and regulate as their child regulates.

This point in the model is also a choice point. If a grownup is unable to connect with how they are feeling and thoughtfully engage with their child, it is often preferable that they don't attempt co-regulation at this point in time. They might be better to leave another grownup to regulate the child or, if it is safe to do so, they may opt to walk away and take some time to regulate themselves a bit more before returning to engage with their child.

O is for Organizing the child's feelings, as well as the situation

As grownups, we have a role in both allowing our children to go and explore and providing nurture when they need it. This second function, which is referred to as safe haven in the Circle of Security model (Hoffman *et al.* 2017), serves the function of nurturing the child and helping to organize their feelings. We often conceptualize children coming to us in sadness; however, children may also come in anger. For many grownups, welcoming a crying child into their arms is something they can readily do, but the child who comes screaming in anger is often much more difficult to welcome in. In both situations, however, what the child needs is for a grownup to help them organize their emotions. In some ways the child who comes in anger may need this more. The child who comes in sadness is connected with that emotion and ready to share it, while the child who comes in anger often needs support to identify the emotions underneath their anger.

Siegel (2012) encourages grownups to "name it to tame it," noting that telling the child the story of their upset supports them to make sense of their experience, using their left brain, and leaves them feeling more in control. Similarly, the Circle of Security model (Hoffman *et al.* 2017) emphasizes the role of grownups being with children, naming their feelings, conveying that these are normal and communicating that they are there to help. The model promotes the idea that grownups need to follow their child's need wherever possible and take charge wherever necessary. Organizing a child's emotions and the situation is about taking charge. The grownup who says "I can see this is too much right now. Would you like to come for a walk with me or should we sit down for a bit?" is organizing both their child's feelings and the situation, doing so in a manner that honors the child's needs whilst gently taking charge.

This process of supporting the child to organize their emotions becomes more difficult as they get older. Their anger can be so spiky and fiery. Often the anger will be directed at the grownup, making it hard to hold and support the child to organize these feelings rather than getting upset and responding in anger. Children can say incredibly hurtful things when they are angry, often unconsciously hitting on those areas that are most provoking to their grownups. It takes a lot to remember that these words reflect the child's distress rather than their actual beliefs or perspective on the situation, and we often have an important role in supporting grownups in this space.

Grownups who have had a moment to connect with their feelings and regulate themselves are much more able to help the child organize their emotions in this context.

They can notice their hurt feelings about what the child is saying or their embarrassment at this occurring in front of family and friends and still support the child to understand and organize their emotions. They can acknowledge the child's anger and demonstrate that they understand where this feeling has come from, helping the child to make sense of what they are experiencing.

In addition to organizing the child's feelings, this step in the model emphasizes the need to organize the situation for the child. Grownups may, for example, say something like "Whoa! This is really too much isn't it? Let's go outside for a moment" and offer children a way to regulate in the moment. This might be about helping them to understand what is happening or finding some way to reduce some of the demand. Siegel (2012) notes the importance of movement in regulation, and this is certainly worth keeping in mind. Moving your body as you go outside, getting a drink of water, having a cuddle or shooting some hoops is very regulating for both grownups and children and is a key aspect of organizing the situation for a child.

Organizing the situation for our children is both proactive and reactive. Proactively, children benefit from understanding what will happen in a given situation. This is particularly true for children who are neurodiverse and find new situations anxiety-provoking. Sometimes grownups also need to organize the situation reactively, in response to noticing that their child is becoming dysregulated. Situations don't always go to plan, and even when grownups have organized the situation proactively, there are sometimes challenges that arise. There can be unforeseen challenges, such as plans changing or long waiting times, or there can be unpredictable elements of a situation that are difficult for the child. For example, a child who is looking forward to receiving a birthday present from a relative might struggle when the present is not what they had hoped. In these situations grownups can respond in a way that organizes the situation for the child, providing structure and options. For example, they might say something like "I know waiting is hard for you and I can see you are getting agitated. Could we color together or would you like to play a game on my phone?" or "This is not going your way and you're feeling really annoyed. Let's both get a drink and then we'll see if we can work this out." In these examples the grownup helps to organize the child's feelings as well as the situation.

Organization is also about limit-setting. Grownups who offer children two choices in a situation are setting limits around what a child may choose. The grownup who offers a child a different way is also setting a limit. These limits are gentle and are accompanied by recognition of, and empathy for, how the child is feeling.

L is for Looking for the feelings underneath

Most grownups are better placed to empathize with and support their child when they understand how their child is feeling. This is particularly true when they are faced with an angry child and notice that they are responding in kind. Knowing that anger is often a secondary feeling and knowing that their child is feeling, for example, anxious, scared, hurt, disappointed or embarrassed can help grownups to connect to these feelings and better support their child in this moment.

Some grownups come to therapy already having a good sense of what their child is feeling, while others need more time and support to do so. Rather than having grownups feel they need to clearly identify the feelings their child is experiencing, the emphasis here is more on the process of considering their child's experience. The empathy that arises when grownups see anger as a sign of distress is what is helpful here, rather than the identification of the specific feelings that might underlie the anger.

Over time grownups begin to learn about patterns for their children, which can help them become much more adept at looking for the feelings underneath. They might notice, for example, that their child is often angry in the lead-up to undertaking something new and understand that there is some anxiety underneath this. Or they might begin to see a pattern of angry outbursts occurring in the evening on days when the family has had a number of social commitments. As grownups begin to hold this awareness of their child, they are often more readily able to predict what will be challenging for their child and can organize these situations more effectively for them, providing greater structure and support as needed.

D is for Doing the things that are regulating

Doing the things that are regulating together with the child might, for some children, mean going for a walk, having a drink of water or snuggling together. Many of the activities in this book, particularly those in Chapter 4, provide an opportunity to explore what is regulating for children. Doing these things together is emphasized in this model, with the knowledge that this is regulating for both the child and the grownup and that as one of them regulates the other will tend to do so as well.

It is worth noting that grownups can find it hard to engage in these regulating activities with their child if they do not understand the rationale for doing so. Many will have been parented with a behavioral approach that utilizes consequences and can feel as though they are inadvertently rewarding the behavior. It is important to talk through these concerns and ensure that grownups understand the role of regulation and know the opportunity to talk about the challenge that will come afterwards.

S is for Speaking after the child and grownup are regulated

In many ways this step in this model is about reflection. Talking helps us make sense of what happened and why; however, not all of this needs to happen with the child. What follows are some considerations around how to navigate this space.

When children are dysregulated, they are not using their thinking brains and cannot be effectively engaged in conversation about what is happening. Despite this, many grownups will endeavor to talk with children about what is happening, assuming that the child is both speaking logically and able to meaningfully comprehend what is said to them. For this reason, the HOLDS model puts speaking at the very end, emphasizing that this should only occur once both the child and the grownup are regulated. Siegel (2012) emphasizes the idea of talking later with his "connect and redirect" strategy, encouraging grownups to connect emotionally with their child and only bring in teaching when the child is more in control.

It is important to note that while we want grownups to hold off on speaking to their child, we do not want them to stop communicating with their child. Indeed, non-verbal communication is essential through the regulation process. Polyvagal theory has highlighted the role that a prosodic voice, a warm and welcoming facial expression and gestures of accessibility have in creating a felt sense of safety (Porges 2017). We want grownups to be engaged and to be communicating non-verbally that the child is safe and supported, valued and loved. Helping grownups to reflect on what they want to be communicating in these moments and reflecting on how they can do so without words can therefore be very helpful.

Exploring how this fits for grownups is important, and the activities included in this chapter can help you to do this. In practice, grownups who tend to regulate themselves by talking often find it hardest to hold off speaking about what has happened. Sometimes encouraging them to engage in reassuring chatter rather than problem-focused discussion is helpful in this space. Providing some information about how long most children take to regulate is often helpful. In my experience, once a child becomes dysregulated it can take 20 to 30 minutes for them to calm. For some children, recovery takes even longer. Grownups who return to talking about the problem too soon often find that children can become dysregulated again very quickly. So, it can also be helpful to support them to recognize the signs that their child is regulated.

Grownups also often find it helpful to know that speaking about what has happened might occur well after the event. They might even choose to talk about it the next day if that is most appropriate for their child. Encouraging grownups to reflect on the purpose of the conversation is often useful. Conversations might help us better understand the child's perspective, allow the grownup to share their perspective, and support the two to problem-solve the situation, identifying what might be different next time. It is important that grownups are realistic about a child's ability to engage in these conversations. Checking in around a grownup's expectations for their child is often helpful. It's important that grownups understand that younger children and those with communication difficulties will be able to engage far less in conversation. Offering examples of what grownups might say in this space is often helpful, noting that this might be as simple as "Next time you get stuck with something you can ask me for help."

These conversations can be a space for problem-solving, but it is important to acknowledge that problem-solving requires a lot of planning and organizational skill. Children continue to develop these skills over time, and grownups often overestimate their capacity in this space. Given this, for most children, I would encourage thinking about one thing that might help or one thing they could do differently next time rather than trying to adopt a model in which all possible solutions are considered and evaluated. Thinking about just one thing is much more developmentally appropriate, realistic and manageable. A simple problem-solving model for children is presented in Chapter 7.

Grownups often have questions about consequences and limits, and these may need to be part of the discussion too once the child and grownup commence this speaking part. Helping grownups to be clear that consequences are for behavior, not for feelings, and ensuring these are not used punitively is important. Encouraging grownups to think about logical consequences can be helpful, and this can often be framed in the context of repair. For example, you might say something to a child like "I get that you were really angry and I'm glad we've got a plan for next time you come home from school so stressed. We are both learning and we'll work this out. I do know though that your brother was very upset and hurt when you hit him, and I'm wondering how you might be able to make that better?" Children might suggest making a card or letting them play with a favorite toy, for example, and grownups can offer similar options, allowing the child to choose between a few if they are unsure. Other examples of repair include fixing something that was broken or tidying up if they threw toys about when angry.

None of these consequences is onerous or extensive, and the child and the grownup can engage in these together. Such consequences enable the child to learn about relational repair and appreciate the impact of their actions, without creating resentment and hostility or causing the child to miss out on important childhood activities. It is important to clarify that I am not suggesting that children be forced to say sorry to others, as there is a risk they will do so in a perfunctory or insincere manner; rather I am suggesting that grownups can provide scaffolding that allows the child to reflect on some of the social implications of their behavior and encourages them to think about relational repair.

As in the examples above, this is a space for problem-solving and negotiation. Siegel (2012) captures it perfectly, encouraging grownups to "engage, not enrage" through asking questions and expressing curiosity rather than immediately listing consequences or other disciplinary action. Indeed, a problem-solving conversation in which a child is encouraged to explore what they might do differently next time is often enough. There are also times when grownups don't need to speak about the problem with their child. For example, a younger child who has language difficulties and has multiple outbursts each day is unlikely to benefit from talking about them.

It is important to note that encouraging repair is not appropriate when children have been traumatized and have become dysregulated because they feel unsafe. In these situations, saying something brief can be helpful, such as "I remember that there was lots of fighting when you lived with your Mom, and I noticed that you got really angry when I told Macy I was frustrated. I do get frustrated at times—however, you and Macy are both safe when that happens. I won't hurt either of you." As in this example, it is essential that the grownup takes responsibility. Older children particularly benefit from acknowledgments such as these; however, what will remain most helpful is repeatedly experiencing safety in this context. Over time, children will learn that they are safe and become less triggered. A consequence in this context, when children are responding in ways that have previously been protective or adaptive, is unhelpful. It also impacts on the relationship between the child and grownup, often doing so at a time when they are still working to establish strong connections.

It can also be helpful for grownups to know that they don't always need to talk about what has happened in detail. Sometimes it is enough to acknowledge that everyone's feelings got too big and that this is something you are all continuing to work on.

Considerations when using this model

Many of the aspects of this model are linked, and families are encouraged to use these strategies flexibly. For example, grownups will often reflect on what their child might be feeling when they connect to their own feelings (Having a moment), looking for those feelings that are underneath the anger their child is expressing (L). Similarly, engaging their child in regulating activities (Doing the things that are regulating) is a way in which the grownup can organize (O) the situation for the child. This generally works well and there is no need to use the steps sequentially; rather the model provides a helpful way of reminding grownups of some of the key aspects of regulation, allowing them to use these flexibly with their child. The one step that is often an exception to this is speaking about the situation (S), which is generally unhelpful when the child and grownup are not regulated.

Some grownups will need more help to work out how they can regulate their child, while others will quickly integrate these strategies. Some will have had the experience of being regulated by loved ones and will have a template for doing so, while others will not have had this experience. Particularly for those grownups who are in the latter category, seeing you regulate the child within sessions and having you support them through this process is often very powerful. Perhaps even more importantly though for these grownups is the way we hold them too, providing a safe relationship in which they feel accepted and understood as we help them to do so for their child. Having a good sense of the grownups you are working with will help you know how they can best engage with this model, letting you know how to pace the way you work with the model and how the family might most effectively engage with it.

Grownups can be invited to lean in to the parts of the model that they find the most challenging and explore what this might be about for them. Ensuring that you support them with this throughout therapy is important. For example, when grownups have not used language around feelings at home and lack a template for this from their own childhood, it is unrealistic to ask them to do this at home until they have been supported to do so in sessions. Similarly, when grownups struggle to tune in to their own emotions, asking them to do so between sessions to begin with is unhelpful. Indeed, asking grownups to do things they are not yet able to do may lead to them feeling further defeated and disengaging from therapy. Rather, we need to support grownups in these spaces, offering lots of opportunity for them to practice this in sessions before suggesting they practice these skills at home.

Grownups can also reflect on aspects that they already do well and, in the case of families that have more than one grownup, on how they might support each other with these various aspects.

When grownups don't get it right

Parenting is undoubtedly the hardest job in the world. No one gets it right all of the time, and we need to have a lot of grace for grownups. It's not possible to be attuned and supportive all of the time, nor is it helpful. The experience of rupture in relationships is normal and it allows grownups an opportunity to repair with children, showing them that people make mistakes and that apologizing and finding ways to make this better allows us to repair relationships. This process is similarly highlighted by Hoffman and colleagues (2017), who note that the process of rupture and repair can be incredibly beneficial to the child. *Rupture and repair with Play-Doh* is an activity included in this chapter that helps grownups and children to know that rupture is inevitable and to remember that repair is possible.

It is also important to recognize that families who come to therapy often face many challenges that other families don't. They may have children who are dysregulated many times each day, which can significantly reduce a grownup's resources and their capacity to respond supportively. Grownups can feel exhausted and worn down and may also start to feel resentful of their child or avoid spending time with them. In turn, children whose grownups respond in this way are likely to become increasingly dysregulated. Often, by the time families come to therapy, many of these patterns are apparent, and acknowledging this complex interplay is sometimes more important than exploring how these challenges first originated. Creating a safe space in which grownups can reflect openly on how they are responding and see where they might be able to change this is valuable. Many of the children we see in therapy will have a level of reactivity or other challenges that make responsive parenting even more crucial.

Supporting grownups to regulate their child effectively outside of sessions is one of the most influential things we can do. Doing this well requires us to hold the space for grownups, acknowledging how difficult this can be, and supporting them to repair the situation when they aren't able to respond effectively. Repair might take the form of a verbal apology or an action and is something we can model with the child and family when ruptures in our relationship with them arise.

When therapists need to use HOLDS

MAX

Max had needed support from his mother and me to regulate throughout the session. At the end of the session he was reluctant to leave and remained seated when his mother and I rose to leave. He did not respond to his mother's encouragement to stand up and became oppositional, refusing to move, and beginning to raise his voice. I had been running over time and needed to pick up my own children so, noticing my own anxiety, I took a breath and grounded myself. I explained to Max that he was my last person for the day and that I needed to leave. I acknowledged that he didn't want to do so and that going from one thing to another sometimes made him feel anxious. I checked in with his mother about the plan for the remainder of the afternoon so Max knew what was coming up. As I did so, I took his shoes, which he had taken off during the session, and untied the laces, loosening these as I did to make it easier for him to put the shoes on his feet. While Max put on his shoes, I again clarified the plan for the afternoon and asked if Max could send me a photo of a toy he'd mentioned once he got home. Max and his mother sent the picture through as soon as they got home.

MAGGIE

Maggie had come in with her sister and parents for a family session. Her sister chose a board game and I noticed some initial anxiety, knowing that Maggie often struggled to regulate herself in games. Maggie was keen to play, however, and I decided I would model some regulation strategies on my turn. Unfortunately Maggie had a turn prior to me and it didn't go her way, causing her to become dysregulated. After regulating her I apologized, saying that I knew games were hard for her and that she was still working on managing the feelings that came up. I suggested a much simpler game which I knew Maggie had managed well in her sessions with me and we chose to play that instead.

The HOLDS model works for therapists too and being able to demonstrate this in our sessions helps the child's grownups to see this in action. In the Max example above I had a moment to notice my own feelings and regulate myself (H), organized the situation for Max (O) by finding out what was coming up after the session and helping with his shoes, and looked for the feelings underneath (L), helping him to organize his feelings by naming that he often feels anxious in this situation. I also supported Max and his mother to think about what they could do (D) by asking them to take a photo when they got home.

Like a child's grownups, we sometimes get it wrong. We might misjudge where a child is at and ask too much of them, leading to an angry outburst. We might offer a calming strategy that is a poor fit and, in doing so, inadvertently cause a child to become even more angry. These situations give us an opportunity to repair the rupture, modeling to the child how we can do so. As in the example of Maggie above, demonstrating this for grownups is also helpful and often reassures them that you have understood how challenging it can be for them. Noticing ruptures and repairing them sooner rather than later is important and highlights again the need for us to be ever present in sessions.

★
Handout: HOLDS for your child

H is for Having a moment to connect with your own feelings and look after yourself

- Take a breath.

- Notice how you are feeling.

O is for Organizing the child's feelings, as well as the situation

- Think about how your child is feeling.

- Gently name this for them (e.g., "It's really upsetting" or "Oh, that is frustrating").

- Organize the situation (e.g., "We need to take a break" or "After this we can look for it together'").

- Set limits as needed.

L is for Looking for the feelings underneath

- Look for the feelings underneath the anger or behavior.

- Connect with these feelings.

- Gently name these feelings (e.g., "I'm wondering if you are worried about the concert tonight" or "It sounds like you felt really left out").

D is for Doing the things that are regulating

- Do the things that are regulating together (e.g., suggest that you both take a break, get a drink of water or go for a walk).

S is for Speaking when you are both regulated

- Talk about what happened only when your child is regulated and able to use their thinking brain.

- Encourage your child to share what they were thinking and feeling.

- Reflect on anything they could do differently next time.

- Help the child to think about repair if need be.

Talk, don't talk

Talking can be helpful; however, grownups are often tempted to talk too much when children are angry. This activity helps children and grownups to explore this tendency and gives them an opportunity to play around with how they might be able to express something without words.

What you need
Toy buzzers that light up and make a sound when pushed or paper and some markers.

Introducing this activity
You can introduce this activity by suggesting that you play a game a bit like charades together. For this activity, I use some game show buzzers I have, suggesting that the child designates one as the *Talk* button and one as the *Don't talk* button. If children are sensitive to sound or if you don't have buzzers available, you can simply help the child to make two signs, one saying *Talk* and the other saying *Don't talk*. This activity is difficult online as you really need to be able to see all of a child's and grownup's body in order for this to work well.

Children are typically very happy to be in charge of the buzzers or signs, which works well, but, if they choose to, the child and grownup can swap roles, each having a turn to communicate the message. We generate the messages together, making sure these are a good fit for the child and family, and writing these on pieces of paper before placing them in a box to be drawn at random. Some example messages are included in the box below, which contains both neutral messages and emotionally supportive ones. The inclusion of neutral messages can be helpful as it provides a contrast to the emotionally supportive messages. Having a mix is particularly useful for children and families who tend to engage in less emotional expression and may find this less comfortable.

To begin playing the game, encourage the grownup to draw out a message from the box. Explain that when you say "Go" they will need to communicate this message to their child, but their child will use the buzzers or signs to decide whether they should communicate this verbally or non-verbally. Let the child know that they can choose *Talk* or *Don't talk* at any point, even when their grownup is part way through a response. This typically creates an element of fun, allowing the child to guess at the message their grownup was trying to send. While the child and grownup are likely to play the game by trying to communicate the message accurately, therapeutically the focus is around reflecting on the ways in which grownups can use soft eyes and a gentle face and body posture to communicate a sense of safety to their children. This is what we want to give children and grownups the opportunity to play around with.

Encourage the family to reflect on what it was like to send the message non-verbally as opposed to verbally. What was it about their face or body that enabled them to communicate effectively? Are there times when non-verbal communication works well for them at home or elsewhere?

Once the family has a sense of this, you can ask them about what form of communication might be best when their child is angry. If the family are unsure, I will often talk here about how when we are really angry we are less able to access our thinking brain and go on to explore this. I might, for example, ask how they know if the communication is working when their child is angry. We might also wonder what are the signs that their child is regulated enough to hear what they are saying. Remembering that each child is different we might wonder what sort of non-verbal communication the child prefers when they are dysregulated.

Considerations and adaptations

Sometimes grownups become anxious when they are unable to speak, and it is important to notice this. This anxiety is often around a grownup valuing the opportunity to talk and express their point of view so it is important to honor this whilst still encouraging the grownup to reflect on when is the best time for talking. The HOLDS model can be used to remind grownups of this.

Examples of helpful messages to try to communicate

Neutral messages:

- It's on the ceiling.
- I can see it under the chair.
- Put it in my pocket.

Emotionally supportive messages:

- You're the best.
- I get this is hard.
- I'm here for you.
- I know you're upset right now.
- You've got this
- It's ok.
- I love you.

Rupture and repair with Play-Doh

This activity helps grownups and children to understand that rupture is inevitable and repair is possible. It is particularly helpful for grownups who have perfectionistic ideas around parenting or those who find it hard to repair after a rupture.

What you need
Some Play-Doh.

Introducing this activity
To introduce this activity, I explain to the grownup and child that I want to explore something I have noticed about relationships. I ask if I can take some Play-Doh out so we can explore this and offer some to the grownup and child, taking some for myself. I suggest that we each try to roll the Play-Doh into the longest sausage we possibly can to show all the time the child and their grownup have spent together, talking about all of the things they do together.

As we roll the Play-Doh, it inevitably breaks at some point, and I use this as an opportunity to talk about how all relationships will have points at which there is a break or rupture like this. We talk together about how this might be a disagreement, a fight or a misunderstanding, and notice some of the ruptures that have occurred in the family. Together with the grownup and child, I will wonder about what we can do to fix this up, which typically prompts a suggestion of squishing the Play-Doh back together. As we do so, we notice that we can continue rolling the sausage again. This provides an opportunity to explore some of the ways in which the child and grownup are able to come back together and repair after a rupture and often prompts some useful discussion. This process can be repeated a number of times to emphasize that any relationship that continues over time will inevitably result in a rupture at some point and will require repair.

Considerations and adaptations
I have described how I use this activity when working with a grownup and child together, but whether you do this with the child present will obviously depend on your clinical judgment about whether this is best for the family. This activity could be completed online if the family have Play-Doh they can use.

CHAPTER 7

THINKING ABOUT ANGER

As we've discussed, children (and their grownups) are unable to engage in cognitive strategies unless they have some level of regulation. For this reason, this chapter comes after those on understanding, co-regulation and calming, positioning these strategies clearly after that work. Some considerations for this work are discussed, along with a discussion of both cognitive strategies and problem-solving.

How and when to use cognitive strategies

RAJ

Raj (10 years) had autism and, despite having good language skills, found it hard to reflect on his feelings and thoughts saying he "didn't know." His father and I worked to notice and name his feelings and supported him to notice some of the shifts that happened when he first began to become dysregulated, such as his voice getting louder and asking for the same thing over and over again. We helped him understand his triggers and put in place environmental changes that reduced the number of outbursts he was having. Raj was supported to develop some more coping skills, and we created some calming tools that he could use both at home and at school, encouraging his father and his teacher to prompt him to use these tools. Raj's angry outbursts decreased significantly. He was still unable to identify the thoughts he had when angry, however he was able to engage in some work around helpful thoughts, generating an "Important things to remember when I am angry" list. This included points such as "Everyone gets angry sometimes," "My angry feeling won't last forever" and "I can use my words to let someone know how I am feeling." This list was shared with his family and school, who were able to use this language with Raj when talking about his anger.

EMILY

Emily was the youngest child in a family of four children. As a preschooler Emily was using words to convey her feelings, expressing her anger and sadness to her parents. This stopped however when Emily was 4 years, around the time her father's mental health rapidly deteriorated. He was irritable and angry and often shouted. Emily became very focused on trying not to upset him and was said to have been hypervigilant around this time. She was referred for therapy at age 7 in the context of concerns about her self-esteem and her lack of ability to stand up for herself in peer interactions. Her father's mental health had improved significantly by this time; however, Emily's presentation suggested she had internalized the belief that anger was unsafe. Consistent with her age, however, she did not convey this directly. Through play she was supported to explore her experiences of anger, and her family began to facilitate safe expression of emotions at home. She gradually became more able to express her feelings and was able to stand up for herself as needed.

During the first sessions, it is helpful to get a sense of how children understand thoughts and what they think about anger. This can guide the way in which you talk about thoughts throughout therapy. For example, if a child has not been able to notice any thoughts in their first sessions, it can be helpful to simply notice your own thoughts as you move through therapy as a way of gradually introducing them to this idea. This can be as simple as noticing your thoughts about what you might do in the session, such as "I'm having a thought about using the sandtray" or similar.

When talking about thoughts in therapy, it is worth thinking about language you use around thoughts. If you are going to use the ACT approach, you are likely to want to model language, such as "noticing a thought"; whereas if you use a more traditional CBT approach, you might use language like "I'm thinking." Using this language incidentally throughout therapy is helpful and might support some children to notice and engage differently with their thoughts. For others, it will lay the groundwork and provide a common language for when you do focus more on cognitive strategies.

One of the other reasons cognitive work is best left to last is that the other work we do often results in changed thinking patterns. This can occur through offering the child and grownups a different way of experiencing situations in the clinic room and changing the patterns of interaction in the family and, as in the examples above, does not always involve addressing cognitions directly. Indeed, this is a core component of CBT: namely that our actions can change the way we think.

This is particularly true when we consider what is referred to as core beliefs in CBT. Core beliefs are those ideas that we hold about ourselves, others and the world. Children are rarely able to articulate these and we generally infer them from their behavior and early history, as in the example of Emily above. The far-reaching nature of these beliefs and the fact that they are rarely articulated in child work means that we often address them through our systemic interventions rather than focusing directly on them. It is through our relationship with the child and family and the way in which we support them to engage with each other and their world that we are best able to influence these broader thinking patterns.

What children are more able to access and talk about is their thoughts in the moment. From around 7 or 8 years of age, children understand what thoughts are and can articulate them. You can get a sense of an individual child's ability to do so during your first session by asking them to add a thought bubble to a drawing and noticing whether they are able to reflect on their own thinking. When children present with angry outbursts, it can be helpful to explore their thinking about anger more generally, about what leads to their anger and about their ability to manage it. Children may for example describe thoughts such as "It's not fair," "Nobody understands," "I can't control this," "I'm just like my Dad" or "It's never ok to get angry." When children can articulate thoughts such as these, and continue to do so when you have helped them to understand anger and develop coping strategies, you might like to use some of the activities in this chapter to work further on this.

Even when children are not articulating uncomfortable or unhelpful thoughts about themselves or about anger, it can be useful to engage in some cognitive work toward the end of therapy. Therapy, it must be remembered, is about developing skills and building capacity as much as it is about reducing symptoms. Developing an awareness of thoughts, therefore, and building healthy thinking patterns is often a good way to build a child's resilience prior to them finishing up the work. For children who have an awareness of thoughts and can engage directly in cognitive work, some of the activities in this chapter can help them to develop their skills in this space. For younger children or those whose development is delayed in this area, we are unlikely to engage them in these activities directly, though we may support their grownups to understand the role of thoughts and be able to model some helpful ways of thinking. As in the example of Raj, we can consider how we can help the grownups around a child to support this work. Similarly, with younger children, we might focus on facilitating different experiences, which in turn is likely to build more balanced thinking patterns, which was the focus of the work in the example of Emily. In the box below are some ideas to pass on to grownups to encourage them to model thinking at home. As always, this is far easier for grownups to do if they have seen you do this in sessions.

Developmentally, children younger than 7 years of age tend to use private speech, speaking words that guide their actions out loud. These ideas later become internalized as thoughts or what might be referred to as inner speech, which is increasingly used in middle childhood (Alderson-Day and Fernyhough 2015). When modeling helpful thinking patterns for younger children, therefore, it is useful to say your thoughts out loud. You can also name their private speech as thoughts. For example, when children say "This is really hard," you might reflect "You're having a thought that this is really tricky." This helps extend a child's knowledge of their own experience and introduces some language around thoughts, helping them to learn more about thinking strategies.

Helpful ways of supporting younger children to understand thoughts and develop healthy patterns

- Notice your own thoughts, labelling them as such—"I'm having a thought that…"

- Share some of your uncomfortable thoughts, where appropriate, such as "I'm having a thought that I'm not very good at gardening…"

- Show your child that you can undertake committed action— "I'm going to keep gardening because it's something we do as a family."

Helpful concepts around thoughts

It is helpful for children to be able to notice their thoughts, to understand what thoughts are and aren't and to know that thoughts come and go. In this section we'll cover some helpful concepts that are useful for children and grownups to understand about the thoughts that arise in moments of dysregulation and anger. Some activities for helping children to explore this are included at the end of the chapter.

The language used around thoughts in this chapter, as well as the selection of strategies, is very much based on an ACT perspective. In practice I find that most children engage well in this space. They can learn that thoughts might be comfortable or uncomfortable, helpful or unhelpful. They can understand that thoughts are just thoughts, that they come and go, and that we can do what is important despite having uncomfortable thoughts. Some children do, however, want to challenge their thoughts, in a more traditional cognitive behavioral manner. If you are working with a child who seems to need this sort of approach, you might like to explore some of the activities in *Creative Ways to Help Children with Big Feelings* (Zandt and Barrett 2017), such as *Kick back soccer*.

One of the concepts that it is particularly helpful for children to understand is the idea of having both a thinking and a feeling brain. First, as noted earlier in this book, the DBT concept of the thinking and feeling brain can be useful for children and is a good introduction to using conscious decision-making. The thinking brain includes the topmost parts of our brain, those that are capable of problem-solving and complex thought. It is what Dan Siegel (2012) refers to as the *upstairs brain*. The feeling brain involves those lower parts of our brain, those that are more primitive, and is referred to as the *downstairs brain* by Siegel. Importantly, both our feeling and thinking brains are important, and we are most effective when we use both, tuning in to our feelings and being curious about what these are telling us before thinking and making conscious choices about this. The concept honors what our feelings tell us, promoting a curiosity around this, whilst still allowing us to use conscious thought and decision-making to choose how we want to respond.

The idea that we want to tune in to what we are feeling *and* be able to make good choices around this is helpful for both children and grownups to understand. This involves reflecting on feelings, rather than responding impulsively "in the integration of head and heart" (Greenberg 2002, p.37). Moments of anger are not the time for making decisions or conversing about the challenges. Rather, regulation is required to enable the child to be able to use both their feeling and thinking brain. The activity *Feeling and thinking brain* in *Creative Ways to Help Children Manage Anxiety* (Zandt and Barrett 2021) is an ideal way to introduce this to children, encouraging children to build a model of the brain using clay. One of the activities featured in this chapter, *Thinking and feeling brain hats*, allows children to explore their feeling and thinking brain, learning more about how each works. The activities *Anger word match* (in this chapter) and *Who's that knocking* (Chapter 5) also connect angry feelings with conscious thinking about what a child might need, encouraging them to use both their feeling and thinking brain.

Another concept that can be particularly helpful for children is understanding what they can and can't do something about. Many children become upset about things that are outside of their control and can become quite angry in this context. While it is helpful to acknowledge what children don't have control over, it is useful to encourage them to think about what they are able to make some choices about. Importantly, this is not about suggesting that children can control their feelings, rather it is about helping children understand that they can choose how they respond to those feelings. The language I find particularly useful with children here is what is "in their hands" and what is "out of their hands," which tends to give them a concrete picture of what they can and can't do something about. Research suggests that adolescents who believe that their emotions are reasonably controllable, experience fewer anxious and depressive symptoms, with theoretical models proposing that this belief prompts the use of emotional regulation strategies (Somerville *et al.* 2023). The *In and out of my hands with anger* activity is a useful way of introducing this to children and the language can be carried through your conversations.

As anger is often a secondary emotion, many children will identify lots of anxious thoughts when they are dysregulated. For some children, cognitive work is a good opportunity to address this anxiety. Many of the activities in this chapter will be helpful for these children; however, *Creative Ways to Help Children Manage Anxiety* (Zandt and Barrett 2021) also includes a section on cognitive strategies that is likely to be useful.

Many grownups find it helpful to learn about these concepts too. They can find it useful to recognize their own thoughts when they become dysregulated, to connect with their own feelings, while still using their thinking brain to make good choices, and to reflect on what is in and out of their control. The latter is particularly helpful to explore in the context of regulating children. For example, while grownups are able to offer calming strategies when regulating a child, they are not able to insist that a child engages with these. While they are able to prepare their child for situations, how situations actually play out is often out of their hands.

Problem-solving

Another cognitive strategy is problem-solving. Many children who have angry outbursts lack problem-solving skills, and teaching these skills can be helpful. Indeed, problem-solving is considered a core element of evidence-based practice for children with behavior difficulties (Garland *et al.* 2008; for a review of its usefulness with children and adolescents, see Kazdin 2017). As with developing healthy thinking patterns, building problem-solving skills is another way of supporting children to develop resilience toward the end of therapy, helping to prepare them for upcoming challenges. Problem-solving can be challenging for children for a number of reasons, which I will explore further. Having a sense of how individual children solve problems is crucial for tailoring your approach in therapy, allowing you to focus on those aspects that a child needs greater support with.

Importantly, the first step in problem-solving is recognizing that there is a problem to be solved. For children who are dysregulated and have angry outbursts, there are two aspects that are worth considering here. The first is the need to recognize that they are angry, which we have explored in previous chapters, and the second is the ability to read social situations (Matthys and Schutter 2021). Some children miss social cues and don't engage in problem-solving because they have yet to perceive that there is a problem. It is often helpful to spend more time helping these children to tune in to the facial expressions and body language of those around them to help them understand that they need to move into problem-solving. You might consider referring a child to a clinician who specializes in social and play skills for support in this space. The problem-solving model utilized in the Coping Power program (Powell *et al.* 2017) emphasizes problem identification as a first step, ahead of encouraging a child to consider their choices and the consequence of each. The model proposed in this chapter assumes that children can identify problems. If, however, children need support to read social situations, focusing on this first is likely to be helpful.

Most problem-solving models involve the child generating strategies, despite our understanding that higher-level cognitive functions are often compromised in times of heightened emotion. Programs that encourage regulation as a first step, such as the Stop Now and Plan program (Child Development Institute 2016), which encourages children to regulate by counting to 10 or taking a deep breath, are likely to be more effective. The model presented below emphasizes pausing and breathing to support the generation of a solution.

Problem-solving models that require children to generate multiple strategies may be difficult to use in a timely way, which is a challenge when a child is facing a problem with a sibling or is angry about something another child is doing at school. Further, the limited research that has been done on problem-solving in children with behavior difficulties suggests that these children generate fewer prosocial strategies than their peers (Matthys and Schutter 2021) and may be more inclined to generate and select aggressive strategies (e.g., Van Rest *et al.* 2020). This suggests that children with emotion regulation difficulties may find problem-solving particularly challenging and requires us to consider carefully what we ask of them in this space. Models that encourage children to choose from a range of options may also imply that there is a correct option. However, we often need to try a strategy a few times for it to work, or we need to try a few strategies prior to finding the right one. Indeed, encouraging resilience is about helping children to recover when something does not work.

Given that children with angry outbursts are likely to need support with many aspects of problem-solving, it is essential that we help create a scaffold for them. Children need support from grownups and teachers as problems arise. They are likely to do best when supported by a grownup who understands the parts they find most challenging and offers suggestions, without solving the problem for them. Indeed, Matthys and Schutter (2021) question whether therapists should engage in problem-solving work independently of grownups and teachers.

On a related note, it is important to remember that seeking help is an effective strategy. In fact, given that many of the children who present for therapy are likely to need a considerable amount of support with problem-solving, this may be one of the most effective strategies we can offer children. For this reason, it is useful to include help-seeking as a strategy when working with children in addition to working closely with grownups and helping them to understand the model so that they can utilize this with the child.

The model below addresses some of these concerns and provides a simpler approach to teaching children to problem-solve. The acronym PIKS makes it easier for children to remember and reinforces the idea that they have a choice. The short and simple nature of the acronym also works well for children who need something basic, particularly in moments of emotion when they have less thinking capacity they can draw on. Some of the activities in this chapter help reinforce this model of problem-solving.

P is for Pausing and taking a breath

Pausing when we notice a problem is an important prerequisite to choosing how we can respond. Helping children to pause for a moment encourages them to act more consciously rather than simply react. The addition of breathing helps children to regulate and puts them in a position to be able to identify a strategy they can use. For children who are familiar with the concept of their thinking and feeling brain, you can explain that this step allows them to engage both aspects of their brain.

I is for thinking of an Idea to try and giving it a go

This step emphasizes the need to think, asking the child to generate an idea. Rather than asking for many ideas, the emphasis is on thinking of one thing that they could try. Implicit in the latter is that the idea must be something feasible: it needs to be something the child actually can *do*. The child does not, however, need to think of more than one idea for what they could try.

When engaging in problem-solving with a child and family, I try to keep the ideas simple and choose ones that can be useful in multiple situations, as this will support the child to be able to use this in their day-to-day living. For example, getting help is a strategy that can be utilized in multiple situations. Younger children will particularly benefit from simple ideas that can be used in multiple situations.

When modeling ideas, it is also important to consider both a child's capacity and their resources. For example, children who struggle with social awareness are likely to need support to navigate social situations, so it might be best for them to seek help from a grownup in this context rather than needing to come up with an idea about how they can manage this on their own. Similarly, if you have been working to improve the way a child relates to their grownup and are wanting to promote co-regulation, ideas such as having a hug with their grownup might be a strategy you suggest.

Encouraging children to try the idea they think of allows them to experience which strategies work and which don't. Implicit in this idea is that they may choose a strategy that is ineffective or unhelpful. For this reason, monitoring is a key element of this model.

K is for Keep going for long enough to see if it works

This step helps ensure children check and see how their strategy is working. Sometimes children will only attempt a strategy briefly; however, some strategies work more quickly, while others take longer to be effective. Walking away from being teased, for example, will either quickly result in the child being able to have some time alone or in being followed and the teasing escalating. On the other hand, however, talking to a teacher about the teasing is likely to take longer, and children need to allow time for the teacher to follow up and talk with the other children before deciding if the strategy has worked. Helping children to understand this concept is often helpful, and you can encourage them to think about how long a strategy they suggest might take to work.

This is also a point at which you can encourage ongoing monitoring as well as inside and outside noticing. Not only can the child notice what is happening around them, such as noticing whether or not the teasing stops, they can also notice what is happening for them. Encouraging children to notice what is happening in their body, how they are feeling, and what their thoughts are is another good way of evaluating whether a strategy has worked. Helpful strategies typically result in greater regulation.

S is for Stop and try something else if need be

This step encourages children to stop if what they are doing is not working and try something else. The idea of trying something else is not necessarily about coming up with a different idea, it might simply be about modifying the idea slightly. Again, this is simpler for children. For example, a child might try walking away only to realize that the child who is upsetting them begins following them, so they may need to modify this by walking toward a teacher. Sometimes it is also helpful to try the same strategy a second time. For example, a child who seeks help from a teacher may not speak loudly enough to be heard the first time and may choose to try a second time, raising their voice a little.

Implicit in the wording of this step is that the action a child chooses may not work. It promotes resilience by helping the child to understand that they can try out an option and try something else if this doesn't work.

Some of the activities in this chapter are aimed at helping children develop their problem-solving skills, and the PIKS model can be used throughout all of these. The model is also summarized in a downloadable handout for children and grownups.

Handout: Problem-solving for kids

Solving problems can be tricky, but you can do it! Here are some steps to help you along the way. Remember you have a choice—you are the one who PIKS!

is for Pausing and taking a breath

- Slow yourself down.

- Take a breath and turn on your thinking brain.

is for thinking of an Idea to try and giving it a go

- Think of something that might help.

- Give it a go.

is for Keep going for long enough to see if it works

- Keep going with the idea you chose.

- Keep noticing if it is working.

- Notice what is happening inside of you as you try. (How are you feeling?)

- Notice what is happening outside of you as you try. (How are others responding? Is the situation changing?)

is for Stop and try something else if need be

- Stop if it is not working.

- Repeat the PIKS steps again.

Lucky dip choices

This is a helpful activity for developing problem-solving skills. It is also useful for reducing anxiety around decision-making, which many children experience.

What you need
A brown paper bag, some popsicle sticks and some markers.

Introducing this activity
I introduce this activity by suggesting to the child that we think about some of the things that could be helpful when they are angry. Depending on the child's cognitive abilities and problem-solving skills, you can decide either to go with what they can do when they are angry or to focus on a situation that the child is having trouble managing. Explain that together you will write some options using markers on some popsicle sticks and place them into a brown paper bag. If you are working online, most families are usually able to find a brown paper bag or even an envelope. If they don't have popsicle sticks at home, encourage them to cut up some strips of paper and use those.

If the child becomes stuck and is unable to think of options, you might ask the grownups, or you could offer a suggestion or two yourself if need be. If the child is unsure about a suggestion, notice gently that they might feel anxious about that idea and encourage them to write it down anyway, reassuring them that they don't have to try any strategies they don't want to. Grownups can be encouraged to make their own bags during the session, and you may also like to make one as a way of modeling some strategies.

When the child has some options in the bag encourage them to give it a name. Children will often come up with something like "My choices when things don't go my way" or "Things that help when I'm angry."

You can then suggest that this is a bit like a lucky dip. The child can choose an option from the bag and won't know what it is. They may or may not like the option; however, if they decide the option is one they want to try, they can do so. If the child doesn't feel like this is a good option for them, or doesn't fit with the situation, encourage them to choose something else out of the bag. Keeping this light and playful reinforces the idea that children can try something and see how it works rather than needing to consider all of the options, consistent with the PIKS model outlined above.

Considerations and adaptations
Practicing with this bag in the session using role play or puppets is often a good way to reinforce the skills. You can also encourage the child to use this bag should moments of anger or frustration arise during the session. Encouraging grownups to consider when a child might need their bag and how children could be prompted to use this is often helpful.

Different roads

This activity allows children to play with the idea of problem-solving, identifying different choices they can make when angry. This is a helpful activity for developing problem-solving skills and supports children to bring a lot of the concepts they have learnt about anger together.

What you need
Paper and markers, blocks and cars or an online map.

Introducing this activity
You can use different materials for this activity, depending on what is most likely to appeal to the child. For example, you might show children who have an interest in technology a map on your tablet or laptop, looking closely at an intersection and talking about the different possible ways you can go from that intersection. Older children may be able to engage in this activity online if you share a picture of a map or draw one on a shared whiteboard. For a younger child or one who enjoys playing with cars, you might use blocks and cars to build some roads and explore some of the intersections you set up. Still other children may prefer to draw a map, which can also be the basis for this activity.

When looking at the intersection with the child it's important to emphasize the decision-making process. For example, if you are driving a car you can pause and look at the roads, wondering about each one you might take. When the child understands the idea of pausing and choosing, you can link this with the idea of making choices in times of anger.

I often say something like "This seems a bit like those times when you get angry. We've been talking about pausing and deciding what you want to do." You may like to identify some of the roads as options the child could choose and link these with concepts the child has worked on previously. For example, you might work together to create a feeling brain road, a thinking brain road and a wise mind road. The child may like to play at driving each of these roads, noticing what this would be like. If they are drawing, they may like to draw a picture of the likely destination at the end of the road. They may like to draw or use blocks to build a street sign that points out the various roads. Street signs can also be made using craft materials. For example, you can make one using a popsicle stick and a piece of cardboard. If you want the sign to stand while you play, you could use a lump of Play-Doh, Plasticine or Blu-Tack as a base.

Considerations and adaptations
In completing this activity, it is important to be mindful of the developmental limitations of problem-solving. Emphasizing pausing and choosing a road to take, with the understanding that you can always drive back and choose another, is often helpful and translates more successfully to the child's day-to-day life. Again, this is consistent with the PIKS model described previously.

Grownups can be included in this activity and encouraged to continue talking with children about pausing and choosing a direction at home. Having something as a useful take-home reminder is a good way to reinforce this. For example, children may like a photo of roads they have built or a screenshot of a map you have looked at. If you have created a street sign pointing out the various roads, this is also a useful thing for them to take home.

Problem-solving puppets

This activity is useful for introducing children to the PIKS model, doing so in a developmentally appropriate way.

What you need
Hand or finger puppets, paper and markers.

Introducing this activity
I often introduce this activity by empathizing with some of the challenges a child is facing and suggesting that we play around with how we can solve problems. I encourage the child to choose a puppet and we enact a problem that is similar to the one they are facing.

Choosing an appropriate moment, I say, "Wow!—I'm really feeling the need for us to pause here. Maybe we need to stop and take a breath?" I then suggest that I write down P for Pausing and taking a breath on a piece of paper so that we can keep a record of the things we do that help. As we move back into the play, I'll notice when an idea comes up, from the child or me, and again suggest pausing and writing this on the page, noting that I is for thinking of an Idea to try and giving it a go. I ask the child about how long we should try the idea for and we note down K for Keep going for long enough to see if it works.

I've noticed that children sometimes stop here in their play, leading to a positive ending once they have chosen and tried the idea. When this happens, we celebrate how well that worked before getting curious about whether there might be times when that strategy does not work. Encouraging the child to engage with me again in play around this, we notice that we need to see if a strategy works and try something else if it doesn't. Again, note this on the page: S for Stop and try something else if need be.

Moving in and out of the play in this manner seems to be more effective than waiting until we have enacted a scenario and writing down each of the steps, which requires more from a child in terms of memory and cognition. The other aspect of doing it in this way is that it models the process of slowing down and consciously thinking: the ability both to be in a situation and to reflect on it.

Grownups can, of course, be readily involved in the puppet play, and I often encourage them to take the role of other puppets, following the child's direction about what they need to do. They can also be encouraged to share about times in which they have observed children engage in each of these steps. If you are working online, you might like to use some puppets and have the child use stuffed toys at their house, noting the steps in the model on the online whiteboard to share with the family afterwards.

Considerations and adaptations
When reflecting on this activity with the family, it is helpful to talk about the acronym PIKS and ask about when this might be helpful for them. It is also useful to ask about how the child can best remember these steps, knowing that it is harder to do so in the moment. The family might like to take the page on which you recorded the PIKS steps home, or you might agree on a way in which the grownup can prompt and support the child through these steps.

Anger word match

This activity helps children to begin thinking about what words might fit for them when they have angry feelings, supporting them to communicate more effectively in this context.

What you need
Cardboard and markers, as well as some puppets.

Introducing this activity
To introduce this, I will say that I've noticed that sometimes our angry feelings prompt us to say something to others. I explain, for example, that we might say if we don't like something or when we want someone to stop doing something. I then suggest that we write some of these words down and see if we can match them to situations. Drawing a speech bubble on an A4 page of paper and writing the words in this is often a good way to do this and should mean that you end up with multiple pages with something the child could say on each. Some words that children might find it helpful to say when they are beginning to feel dysregulated are listed in the box below. It is important, however, that the words you identify should be developed collaboratively, holding in mind the needs of the individual child and family. It is important to ensure that the language you choose is also developmentally appropriate for the child.

> **Helpful things children might be able to say when they are becoming dysregulated**
>
> - I'm finding that annoying. Could you please stop?
> - This is making me uncomfortable.
> - I need some time on my own right now.
> - I'm feeling overwhelmed and need a break.
> - Please leave me alone.
> - Stop it—I don't like it.

Once we have generated a number of speech bubbles, we can enact some situations and encourage the child to match these to one of the speech bubbles. How you choose to enact this will depend on the child. Younger children often enjoy puppets, while I find older children enjoy using a clapper board and playing the role of director. If you are working online you might like to use the child's soft toys or have them mime a clapper board action with their hands while you enact some scenarios with puppets.

Considerations and adaptations

Some children will readily provide examples from their lives and enact these; others will need some distance from this and may need you to use your clinical knowledge to enact scenarios with some similarities, whilst still ensuring they feel safe by drawing on the distance that play provides. Either way, pausing and encouraging the child to think about which words fit in the scenario is helpful. If you are working online, you might encourage the child to bring out some of their stuffed toys to enact the scenarios and you can draw the speech bubble on the online whiteboard, sharing it with the family after the session.

When reflecting on this activity, it is useful to encourage the child and their grownup to think about what sorts of words their anger might prompt. Grownups might share about some of the helpful words their own anger prompts or may give examples of when a child has been successful in using their words. Supporting the family to think about this and wondering together how the child might be reminded of these words is helpful. The family may like to take home a speech bubble with words that are a good fit for them and display it somewhere as a reminder.

Sticky thoughts with sticky tape

This activity is useful for those children who get caught up in thoughts that make them angry, such as "It's not fair." The activity provides a way of exploring how these thoughts might get in the way of what they want to do. Because this activity focuses on thoughts, it is appropriate for older children who can recognize and articulate their thoughts.

What you need

Masking tape (wide enough to write on) and some markers. You will also need some activities that the child enjoys completing.

Introducing this activity

I like to introduce this activity when I am engaged in drawing or playing a puzzle or game with the child. I then begin naming some thoughts that come up for me as we play, such as "I'm having the thought that I'm not going to win" or "I'm having a thought that my drawing is terrible." I then reflect on how some of these thoughts are really sticking around and suggest that we write some of these down so we can better think about what is happening, bringing the masking tape out as I do so. I show the child that I can write each sticky thought on a piece of tape and stick it to my finger. I end up with several pieces of tape hanging off the ends of my fingers as I demonstrate this. I then ask about any thoughts that are coming up for the child and encourage them to do the same with their thoughts. I then suggest that we keep on playing and see what happens. As we play, we notice what it is like to draw or play with those thoughts and reflect on how they get in the way. We notice and name the frustration and annoyance and can model and prompt regulation strategies as needed.

There are often some lovely moments of laughter and connection in this context, and children will sometimes want to get rid of the thoughts. At some point, if the child has not yet done so, I will suggest that we perhaps move the thoughts to our sleeves, the table next to our drawing or even the leg of our pants. We continue drawing or playing, again noticing what this is like to have the thoughts still there though less central. Afterwards, we reflect together on times when a child's thoughts get in the way and might add to their anxiety or anger. Some children might remain focused on the drawing, puzzle or game and, if so, we might notice together that the thoughts simply begin to loosen and fall off as we continue playing and no longer focus on them. Again, this can be a really important reflection for children, and you can help them to relate this to some of their other experiences.

Considerations and adaptations

This activity can also be useful for grownups, particularly if they are getting caught up in worried thoughts when their child is angry. You can encourage them to name the "what if" thoughts that come up for them in this situation, writing each on a piece of tape and sticking them on their fingers. You can then ask them to imagine what it might be like to try to connect with their child with all those thoughts on their fingertips. Explore whether they would be able to effectively hug their child or soothe them by rubbing their back. Wonder together about what the experience might be like for their child if they are caught up in these thoughts. When you have reflected on this, you can together wonder about whether there is somewhere less intrusive that you might be able to put the thoughts. For example, could the grownup place the thoughts on their sleeve to enable them to better soothe their child? Could they stick the tape on their leg allowing their hands to be free? The focus here is not on getting rid of the thoughts, rather it is about understanding how this impacts our focus and considering what we might want to focus on instead.

Staying present with their child is difficult for many grownups, and this is a good way of opening up that discussion and exploring strategies they can use, such as breathing, to ensure they can remain focused on their child. Because this activity requires naming uncomfortable thoughts that relate to their child, I would suggest doing this with a grownup in a separate session rather than with the child present.

Some older children will be able to engage in this activity online, and you may like to ask them to have masking tape and scissors ready ahead of time to enable them to do so.

Following this activity, grownups can be encouraged to talk with their children about any 'sticky thoughts' they might be experiencing as challenging situations arise. They can encourage the child to continue doing what is important to them despite the thoughts, knowing that the thoughts will often slowly peel off when they do. Grownups can also begin noticing their own sticky thoughts and can be encouraged to begin to recognize those that tend to stick regardless of the situation, such as "I'm a terrible Mom."

Thinking and feeling brain hats

This activity supports children to explore the idea of using their thinking and feeling brain, allowing them to do so in a playful manner.

What you need
Paper bowls (the kind that are used for picnics) and markers.

Introducing this activity
When introducing this activity, you will need to adapt the explanation you provide both to the child's developmental level and to the content you have previously covered with the child. For example, if you have previously talked about the different parts of a child's brain, you can say that you thought you might explore the thinking and feeling brain further by making some thinking and feeling brain hats. If, however, you have yet to talk with a child about their feeling and thinking brain, you will need to explain about the feeling and thinking brain first. I usually say that the feeling brain is the part where we feel our emotions and that it is really important, but that we can't use our thinking brain when the feelings are too big. I explain the thinking brain, saying that it helps us make choices and solve problems. Once the child understands this, I suggest that we make some hats to explore this further.

I suggest that we use the bowls as hats and encourage the child to write FEELING on one bowl and THINKING on the other so that we can use these to play around with the idea of using our thinking and feeling brains. Choosing something that fits with the child's level of understanding and their experiences, I then go on to give an example. I might, perhaps, choose to explain about a time when I lost a game and felt angry, placing the feeling hat on my head and describing some of the feelings I had in my body. Then I might take a breath and place the thinking hat on my head over the feeling one, explaining that I took a breath and chose to say, "Oh that's frustrating. Maybe I'll win next time."

I might then ask the child to demonstrate a scenario, using role plays as we work together to explore what happens when we use our feeling brain as opposed to our thinking brain. When role playing, you can bring in your previous work together, helping the child to create this connection. For example, you might link this to how their body feels, the actions they tend to engage in, the thoughts that go through their mind and how others might respond.

Considerations and adaptations
Another way to use this activity, particularly if the child does not like engaging in role play, is to engage in play activities during the session and notice when you are using your feeling or thinking brain, donning the appropriate hat when you do so. With some children, you might just model this initially, wearing the appropriate hat as you notice for yourself, before inviting them to choose the hat that fits for them currently.

Using this activity, we communicate that both the feeling brain and the thinking brain are important. We want to listen to what our feeling brain tells us and use our thinking brain to make good choices about what we do with this information. Ensuring that you validate the child's feelings and invite them to be curious about what those feelings are telling them is therefore very important. This can often lead to children rapidly swapping hats or realizing that they are needing both and placing both on their head, which can be a great discovery.

From a DBT perspective, using both the feeling and thinking brain is often referred to as *wise mind*. For younger children, you don't necessarily need to introduce this concept, and it can be preferable to stay with the idea that we just need to use both our feeling and thinking brain. Older children, however, may find the concept of wise mind useful and can engage well with this. This activity can be used to explore this by talking about wise mind as those times when you are wearing both hats or by making another hat to signify wise mind.

If you are working online, you can have some paper bowls handy and can demonstrate over the screen. Checking if the child has any paper bowls they can use at their end can also help. Most families will have plastic bowls in different colors, and you can readily identify one as a feeling brain hat and one as a thinking brain hat if you can allocate a color for each. Another alternative, depending on the online software you use, can be to add different accessories to your face on the screen so that you can choose something to indicate when you are using your thinking brain and something to indicate when you are using your feeling brain.

Grownups can be encouraged to share times they've noticed their child using both their feeling and thinking brain and may be able to provide examples from their own lives. Encouraging the family to take the hats away and thinking about how they might use them at home can be helpful. For example, you might be able to ask that families use the hats when talking about a challenge that has occurred, or the family might choose to place these somewhere in the house as a reminder to everyone to use both their feeling and thinking brain.

In and out of my hands with anger

Children with emotional regulation difficulties often get upset about things that are out of their control. Helping children and grownups to explore this idea can be useful in therapy, and this activity provides a hands-on way of doing this using a game of Uno.

What you need
A deck of Uno cards.

Introducing this activity
Most children are familiar with the game of Uno, which is a game that includes elements of both strategy and chance. Players have choice about how and when they place cards, with their skill in doing so influencing the game. There is, however, also a significant amount of chance with the cards they draw from the deck and the cards the other players place, adding an element of unpredictability. Games such as this are a useful metaphor for the idea of control, which I often talk with children about as being what is in and out of our hands.

I typically introduce this by suggesting a game of Uno. As you play, try noticing and naming the processes about what is in and out of your hands. For example, making comments like "I've got two cards I can choose from now. This choice is in my hands" or "Oh no, I really didn't want that card. I had no choice about what I was picking up." Notice too, how the child responds to moments when they have control and moments when they don't. Reflect on any emotions that come up during the game play and how these relate to the idea of what is in and out of the child's hands. It is really useful to include grownups in the game too, noticing and reflecting as you would for the child.

Depending on the child and where you are at in the therapy process, this may be a good time to also model some regulation strategies. For example, you might name a feeling and take a breath, saying something like "Oh this is so frustrating, I only had one card left and now I have to pick up four! Oh well—hopefully I get some good cards." Consider when doing so what you are modeling for the child, making sure it is developmentally appropriate for them. For example, in this example the child hears the clinician name the emotion, take a breath to calm their body and use a helpful or coping thought. Younger children might, for example, benefit from having more body-calming strategies named for them, while older children might find some of the helpful thoughts more useful. Some children will need more direct support to regulate during the game, so this can be a good opportunity to help grownups to co-regulate children, offering what they need to work through their anger in the moment.

Reflecting after this activity, you can notice patterns that were apparent during the game and link these with the child's day-to-day life, talking about what is in and out of their hands and how they can look after themselves when things are unpredictable or out of their control.

Considerations and adaptations

Older children can manage to play Uno online if they have a deck at home. To do so you need to each shuffle your deck and hold up the card that you are playing so that you are both aware of what you need to match.

CHAPTER 8

CHOOSING AND DOING WHAT IS IMPORTANT

AYDIN

Aydin would often become enraged when he lost in games at school. He would shout and storm off and accuse others of cheating. Aydin was keen to manage this better as his friends had started to avoid playing with him. He identified that it was important to him to be supportive of his friends and chose a figure to represent this. Holding on to this figure as he played a game with the clinician reminded him of what was important to him and helped him to engage in some calming strategies as he played so that he could support others while playing. Practicing this in sessions resulted in Aydin being able to play with other children at school more successfully.

One of the most helpful things that children can learn to do is to work toward what is important to them. Values-based work is a key component of ACT; however, it often seems to be missed by therapists who are working with children. While children are still developing their values, they do have a sense of what is important to them, and phrasing the question in this way often helps. Another option is to talk about what matters to them, which is the language adopted by Tamar Black (2022) in her helpful book *ACT for Treating Children*. In this chapter some considerations around using this approach with children are discussed, and some activities for supporting children with this are included. I've also shared some thoughts here about helping grownups to focus on what is important to them.

Choosing and doing what is important for children

It can be helpful to notice what is important to a child during your first sessions. For example, you might say "It sounds like your friends are really important to you." Thinking broadly about what is important to the children you work with is often helpful. There are children for whom gaming is a true passion and, whilst this clearly is not what we would think of as a value, it is something that is genuinely important to them and is worth recognizing as such. Where possible, it is helpful to explore what it is that children enjoy and see if you can understand the elements here of what is important to them. For example, some children love gaming because it allows them to build and create in a way that they used to with Lego at a younger age; while others love gaming because it provides an opportunity to connect with others and work alongside peers. When these aspects can be drawn out, it is possible to think about other ways in which children might be able to do what is important to them. A child who enjoys the creative element of gaming, for example, may also enjoy having some new more challenging Lego sets. Rather than being around replacing what is important to a child, this is about extending it and finding additional ways to meet this need.

While some children will talk readily about what is important to them, others will need us to become curious about this and explore this further. They may need us to gently offer some suggestions based on what we notice, particularly if their lives have become problem-saturated and what is important to them has become lost. Others will be aware of their interests and values, though will need an invitation to bring these into the space. They may assume that your role is to help with their anger and that you are unlikely to be interested in them more generally.

Beginning to introduce some language around what is important to the child allows them to bring this into the space and provides an opportunity for you to explore how the challenges they are having with anger might get in the way of what is important to them. Perhaps most importantly, however, this approach conveys a respectful and accepting stance in which you can position yourself as supporting the child in what is important to them. Children might, for example, identify that their angry outbursts sometimes get in the way of them spending time with their friends. Being able to articulate this helps a child to understand the role of therapy and increases the likelihood that they will engage in the process.

Choosing what is important is also helpful as you move into more cognitive work with children, helping to support their choice-making and problem-solving. In this space children can be encouraged to move toward what they view as important and identify those choices that resonate with them. Indeed, the activities in this chapter draw out children's values in the context of helping them to make decisions that support this.

Maintaining an emphasis on moving *toward* what is important to us helps children appreciate that the actions we take are no guarantee of success. Rather, our actions are simply a step in the direction that is right for us.

And for grownups

MAY

May valued flexibility and there was no clear rhythm at home: meal times varied greatly as did the time she would put the children to bed. I was curious about whether her children were similar and how this might work for them. Through our discussions May was able to share that the children seemed to value predictability and noted that the evenings were associated with a lot of angry outbursts, particularly early in the evening. May began to create more of a rhythm after school, feeding the children at some point between 6.00 and 7.30pm and following this with some wind-down time prior to bed. The children did indeed value this predictability, and the angry outbursts decreased a little, which allowed us to explore some of the other triggers more readily.

The idea of values-based parenting has been talked about in the context of ACT, with a number of studies exploring this approach with parents of children with autism (e.g., Holmberg Bergman *et al.* 2023). In my practice I find this approach very helpful when working with grownups. Encouraging grownups to reflect on what is important to them when parenting and supporting them to work toward this is collaborative and respectful. Škėrienė and Jucevičienė (2020) recently shared a model integrating values into problem-solving, suggesting that values are important both when deciding on the end goal and when considering alternative approaches. Engaging grownups in working toward what is important to them and finding approaches that fit with their values can be helpful.

Noticing values early in therapy can be useful, and these will often come up through conversation with grownups in the first few sessions. It can be helpful in this context to name these, saying something like "It sounds like learning is important to you" or "I can hear that you value being able to spend time together." Sometimes grownups are not explicitly aware of their values, and helping them to be more conscious of these can lead them to a better understanding of some of the feelings they have about their child's behavior. For example, a grownup who values learning is likely to be particularly upset by a child who becomes anxious and angry in response to small mistakes and does not persist when tasks become difficult.

Reflecting consciously on values also helps grownups identify some of the conflicts that might be arising for them around this. As in the example above, what a grownup values might sometimes be different to what is important to their child. In these situations highlighting the challenge often supports the family to find a way through this. For example, a grownup who values spontaneity might be able to see how important sameness is to their child and may decide to attend last-minute activities alone, only expecting their child to join them for those they have had more warning about.

When there are conflicts around how grownups respond to a child's anger, it is often particularly helpful to recognize that there may be different values that underlie this. For example, a grownup who values independence and resilience may be reluctant to offer comfort when the child is distressed, while a grownup who strongly values nurture and connection may find it hard to allow space for a child to manage their own challenges. Exploring grownups' own values and early experiences in this space is often more effective than simply providing behavioral solutions. When grownups better understand why they each tend to respond the way they do, they are often more able to find a way through this.

As with children, it is important to communicate to grownups that while our values guide us, we will often fall short of our aspirations. Parenting is challenging, and we always need to approach grownups with an accepting and empathic stance, supporting them to be kind to themselves and repair with their children when they need to. The activity *Rupture and repair with Play-Doh* (Chapter 6) helps explore this idea, as does the *Route recalculation* activity below.

Heading toward what is important

This activity is a helpful way to encourage choice-making that fits with what is important to the child.

What you need
A compass or a compass app as well as some toys you can hide. You may also like to use a copy of the template on the next page and some markers.

Introducing this activity
I introduce this to the child and family by showing the compass to them and chatting about how a compass offers direction. You can then suggest that you experiment with this by hiding something, such as a soft toy, in the room and showing the child and grownups how you can use the compass as a source of direction when finding this. To do this, ask the child to look away while you hide something and hide the toy, noting the direction it is hidden in using the compass. Then give the child the compass and explain where they can find it, saying something like "It's 10 steps to the north." Younger children are likely to need more help with the compass and will also benefit from more specific instructions. Older children, on the other hand, may find it more interesting and challenging to have instructions with multiple steps. Younger children may also need more support to reflect on what is important to them.

Once you have spent some time playing with the compass and the child is familiar with how the compass works, you can begin to talk about how this is a bit like making decisions. What is important to us guides the direction we take and the choices we make. Give the child an example by saying something like "Being kind is important to me, so when someone upsets me I try to find a kind way to let them know." Grownups can also be encouraged to share some examples. When they have done so you can encourage the child to think about what is important to them and how this relates to the choices they make.

Children can be invited to use the template below, listing something that is important to them as a reminder of what might guide their decisions.

Considerations and adaptations
Older children who have some awareness of how a compass works can often be engaged in this online. You can share the template in your session and color and complete it as you talk through the activity.

This activity can also be useful for grownups who want to use their parenting values to guide their interactions with their children. Emphasizing that the compass provides us with a direction we can aim for, without implying that doing what is important to us is simple or that we will always get it right, is helpful.

Encouraging grownups to notice when a child makes choices that fit with what is important to them is often beneficial. You can also encourage them to notice when they parent in a way that fits with their own values.

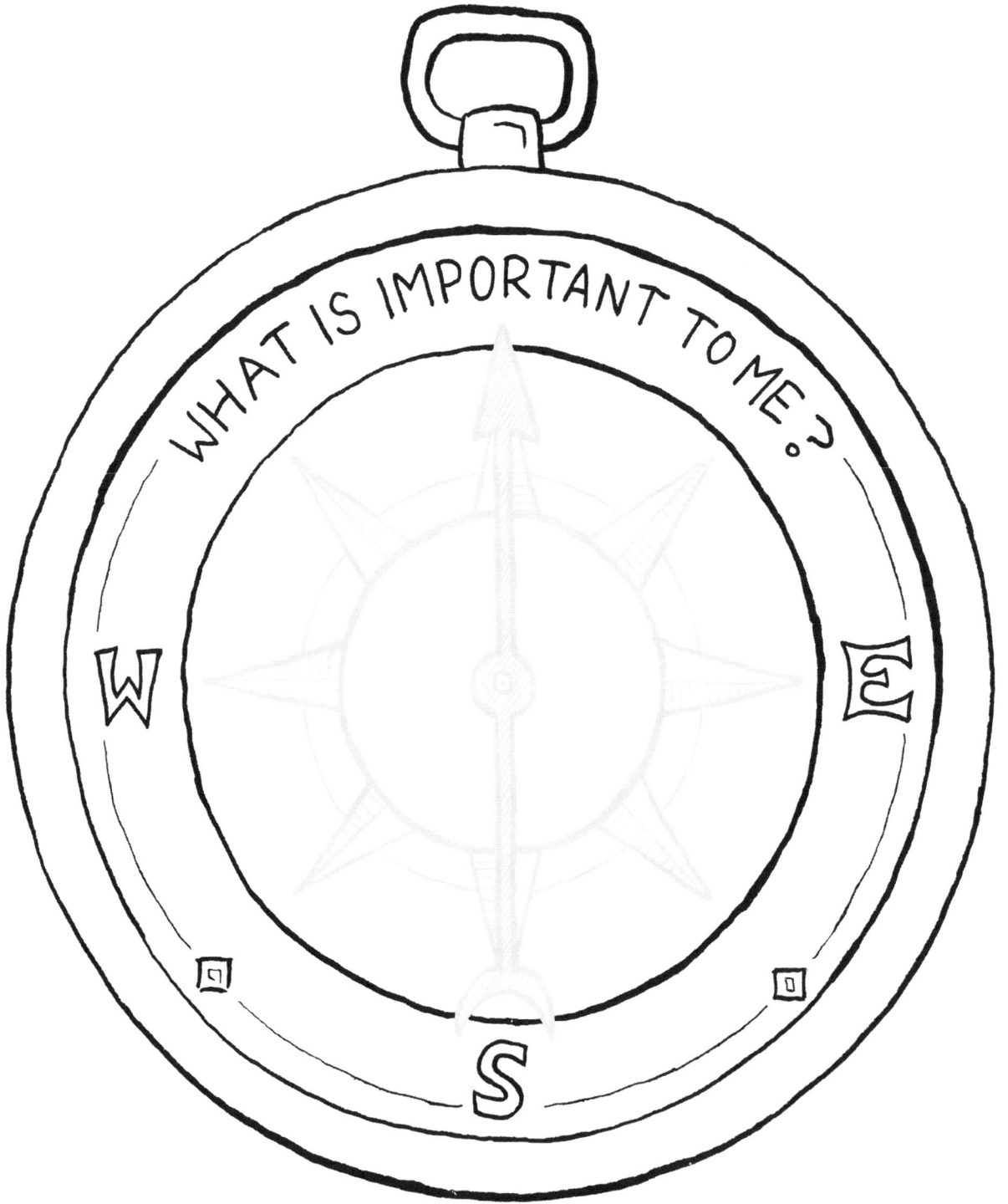

Holding on to what is important

This activity is useful for helping children and grownups think about what is important in a given moment and act upon that.

What you need
Some symbols, toys and figures that the child can choose from as well as some craft supplies.

Introducing this activity
When introducing this activity, I often comment on some of the things I've already learnt about the child, such as that family is important to them, and express a desire to learn more about what really matters to them. You can give some examples of values here and use whatever language fits best with the child and family, whether that be about what is important to them or what matters to them. Children will vary greatly in what they reflect on and may for example identify their pets, playing sport or being a good friend as being important to them. Welcoming whatever they identify as important to them and encouraging them to talk more about it is often helpful. When the child has identified something that is important to them you can ask them to see if there is anything in the room that might remind them of that or whether you should make something together. For example, a child who has identified that caring for animals is important to them might select a small dog toy while a child who loves to spend time outside might choose a stone.

Making something to represent what is important to them is often a good option for children who choose values like being kind or learning new thing or for those children who enjoy crafting. You can for example write, draw, or paint something that is important to the child on a stone or card. You can also use a blank keyring, the kind which are available at craft stores, and decorate it to represent the thing that is important to the child.

Once the child has selected or made something to represent what is important to them encourage them to hold in in their hands. Prompt the child to notice how it feels to really focus on what is important to them. You can then encourage the child to think about what they would do if they were focused on what is important to them. Children may find it hard to come up with examples, so you might need to provide some. For example, you might share that learning is important to you so often read books about child therapy. Support the child to think about times where they act in ways that are consistent with what matters to them. For example, you might identify that a child walks their dog because caring for animals is important to them.

Once the child understands this idea you can encourage the child to apply this to situations they are finding hard. For example, you might have a child who has identified being a good friend as something that matters to them hold onto the object they have selected to represent this while thinking about how they can still be a good friend on the football field when they are feeling upset and frustration about losing the game.

Suggest to the child that you practice what it would be like to get angry while holding on to what is important. You can act out scenarios to explore this. Sometimes children will prefer to have you act out the scenario, and, if so, they can be encouraged to take the role of director, letting you know what you should do. Other times, they might like to do the acting and can benefit from you pausing the play and being curious about whether the option they are choosing is allowing them to hold on to what is important while they are angry.

Considerations and adaptations

Grownups can readily be involved in this activity and can create their own list of what matters to them. They too can choose something in the room to symbolize this and can be encouraged to think about how they can hold on to what is important when they are angry.

Older children can be encouraged to pause and reflect on what is important to them when they become dysregulated. Younger children will need the support of grownups to do so. Helping grownups to reflect on this when supporting their children can be helpful. For example, we might encourage a grownup to share something like "That was really hard and I can tell you are mad. I also know you love playing with Emily. Let's have a cuddle and then you can go play again."

Talking with older children and grownups about how they can practice holding on to what is important even in times of anger is often helpful. It can also be useful to reflect on times when this might be easier or harder and to think about how the child could use what they have made as a reminder of holding on to what really matters to them.

Route recalculation

This activity is useful for helping children to think about what is important to them and work toward this. It emphasizes the need to reorientate in the face of setbacks.

What you need
Paper and markers.

Introducing this activity
As someone who lacks a sense of direction, I have a love-hate relationship with my satellite navigation system. "Route recalculation" is a phrase I hear often and is a great reminder that there is more than one way to get somewhere: ultimately, that the number of U-turns you make does not prevent you from reaching your goal. To introduce this activity, I ask about the child's experience of using a map or of seeing their grownups use one. I then suggest that we draw a rough map outlining the route from their home to the clinic. We often involve the grownup in this process.

Once we have a map drawn, I ask about whether there are any roadworks or detours along the way. If there are, we draw these on the map together and get curious about alternative routes. I share about times when I have been detoured and how I am able to find another way.

Once the child understands this idea I suggest that having somewhere you want to go is like working on something that is important to you. We can then talk about what is important to the child and wonder about some of the setbacks and detours they have faced in moving toward this. Throughout I emphasize that setbacks and detours are to be expected, and I share examples of this. For example, I note that whilst it is important to me to treat others with kindness, I'm not always able to do so and often I have to find a different route or go back and make it better when I don't. We explore what this might mean for the child and normalize their experience, noting for example that they are still likely to shout sometimes. We talk together about what it means to keep our eyes on our destination, remembering what is important to us.

Considerations and adaptations
Younger children are likely to find the higher-level thinking in this activity difficult. It is one that can, however, be useful with grownups. Encouraging grownups to view their own responses as attempts that may take them toward or away from the parenting destination they are aiming for and normalizing the experience of needing to find another way or go back and repair can be helpful.

In reflecting with the family, we talk about how we can remember that setbacks are part of life and how we can be kind to ourselves, knowing that we will continue to move toward our goal. Taking the map home is often a useful reminder of the discussion for children.

Toward ladders and away from snakes

This is a useful activity for helping children identify what they want and reflect on what moves them toward or takes them away from this. When children are angry they often act in ways that move them away from what they want and need rather than toward it. For example, a child who is seeking connection with peers may lash out when they feel left out only to find this isolates them further. This activity draws on the concept of toward and away moves, which is central to ACT. Consistent with ACT, this activity helps children center on what they want and how they can move toward it.

What you need

A piece of cardboard with a grid drawn or printed on it (with squares large enough for a game board), tokens or game pieces, a dice, and some markers. Alternatively you can use a commercially available Snakes and Ladders game.

Introducing this activity

I often begin by asking the child if they know the game Snakes and Ladders. We talk about what the goal of the game is, and I suggest that it's sometimes like life: we work toward something we want or something that is important to us, and there are things we do that move us toward our goal (such as those times we get a ladder) and times when we move away from our goal (a bit like the snakes). We draw the game board together and, as we add ladders and snakes, reflect on those things that move us toward what is important to us and those things that take us away.

Once the game has been created, we can play together using the game tokens and dice. As we play the game we name something that is a toward move when we land on a ladder and an away move when we land on a snake. I will often choose to share something that I am working on to allow me to model this for the child on my own turn. Grownups can also be encouraged to have a turn and to reflect on things that they are working on. They can also share what they have noticed about what the child does that moves them toward or away from their goal if the child needs support with this.

Using a commercially available Snakes and Ladders board game saves time and may be a good choice for children who do not enjoy crafting. It does, however, mean that the child is unable to take this home, so you might choose to share a photo of the board along with a small comment such as "I'm going to remember that one of your ladders is asking for help."

Considerations and adaptations

If you are working online, you can play an online version of Snakes and Ladders with the child.

Younger children will obviously need more support to identify what is helpful and unhelpful, and will need you to keep the language simpler for them. Focusing the game on one thing that is important to them rather than on a broader value often helps. For example, younger children might focus on being a good friend as they play, while an older child might focus on something broader, such as being a kind person. Younger children might need support to reflect on what they can do that helps with this and what doesn't as they land on ladders and snakes. You can encourage them to think of specific examples, such as the time they asked what their friend wanted to play or a situation in which they walked away when angry, noting that these actions are likely to be helpful again in future.

Reflecting with the child and family about how they can make toward moves in their day-to-day life is helpful.

CHAPTER 9

WHEN THINGS GET TRICKY

GRACE

Grace (12 years) became very anxious and would act out aggressively when she was faced with uncertainty or change. She had previously been diagnosed with autism and an intellectual disability. While she had previously been quite settled, some changes in the family had caused her to escalate and she became quite aggressive at home. Her father, who had previously managed this behavior by asking her to go to her room and calm down, attempted to pick her up and move her into her room despite her now being as tall as him.

Anger and aggression are obviously associated with risk. Children who are angry are at risk of hurting themselves as well as others. Furthermore, grownups who are angry are at risk of hurting their children. Aggression in children is also associated with family violence and can signal the need to explore further what is happening in the family. As therapists, we need to be mindful of these risks and evaluate them in an ongoing way. Some considerations are included in this chapter.

Children who are physically aggressive are at risk of unintentionally hurting others as well as themselves. For example, the child who throws or breaks things when angry may unintentionally hurt others. Similarly, grownups who attempt to physically restrain or remove their children may also hurt them. In the moment, when everyone is heightened, the risk of harm is high. Helping children and grownups to understand this and identify safe ways they can manage in this situation is a priority.

There is also a risk that children and grownups will act impulsively when angry, hurting each other and themselves. This risk is often greater when there is a history of impulsive behavior or responding. Understanding the dynamics of how this plays out in the family is important, and it is useful to put some time into planning how the family can respond in times of heightened emotion. Sometimes one grownup within the family regulates themselves more effectively and is therefore a resource in times like this. Sometimes there is a grandparent or similar who acts as a circuit breaker. Being aware of these resources is often helpful.

There is also a chance that when children present with anger issues there is a background of family violence. As discussed previously, studies have shown that emotional dysregulation in childhood is associated with child abuse (Gruhn and Compas 2020; Lavi *et al.* 2019), so keeping this in mind is essential. Creating a safe space for both children and their grownups increases the likelihood that they will share their experiences with us and is, again, a prerequisite for all the work that we do. Therapists who need support in screening for and responding to allegations of family violence are encouraged to seek out further training in this space.

As therapists, we need to be always mindful of these risks, monitoring them throughout therapy. Helping the child and grownups to develop regulation skills is essential, as is avoiding or minimizing anything that tends to escalate the situation.

Developing a plan

Once you have a good understanding of a child's anger and understand the family system, it can be helpful to develop a plan. Explaining to families why it is important to have a plan is a good first step. For example, it can be helpful to explain that anger tends to catch, impacting those around the child and making it harder for everyone to use the thinking part of their brain, making it difficult for everyone to remember how to manage this. In this context the situation can readily escalate and coping strategies can be easily forgotten, which makes having a plan that outlines how everyone can respond in the moment useful.

It is essential that any plan is developed in collaboration with the child and family, using their language. A carefully articulated plan acknowledges the child's anger and explores the meaning of this, with an emphasis on how they can work together to support the child when their anger gets too big. Teachers or other relevant professionals might also be included in developing a plan. A plan can create a bridge between therapy and the child's day-to-day life, building a shared narrative about what happens when the child gets angry and helping others to provide the scaffolding a child needs outside of the therapy room. This means that each child's plan is different, making it hard to use a proforma. Beginning with a blank page conveys clearly to the child that this plan is unique to them and them alone and invites contribution, rather than restricting it.

Involving the child in creating a plan is important. Obviously, children who are older and more verbal can be engaged more in this process, while younger and less verbal children will require further support to do so. What is important, regardless, is that this is approached in a respectful way that communicates to the child that their feelings are acceptable, that they are working on expressing these in an appropriate way and that the grownups around them are going to try to help. Positioning grownups as a support team reduces the likelihood of the child taking an oppositional view of this process and increases the child's sense of autonomy and choice. Prioritizing the child's point of view throughout ensures they are central to this process, increasing the likelihood that they feel connected to the plan.

A plan should provide some documentation around early warning signs and triggers, assisting the child and the adults around them to recognize the anger early. This is articulated in child-friendly language, which is developmentally appropriate, such as "When I start to get angry I..." and "Things that tend to make me angry are..." Carefully articulating what the child and others can do when their anger gets too big is a useful process. It draws all of their strategies together and provides a point of reference for both the child and their grownups.

As discussed, children often need their grownups to co-regulate them when their anger gets too big, and having a written plan can support this. It allows grownups to recognize what is happening, often enabling them to do so earlier than they typically would, which means they are in a much better position to offer co-regulation. Furthermore, the plan offers some suggestions for how co-regulation might occur, reducing the need for thinking and planning in a moment of high emotion. For example, the calming options listed might be things that grownups are needed for, such as having a quiet hug on the sofa, or things they can prompt the child to do, like going and jumping on the trampoline.

Any written plan will need to change over time as therapy progresses and the child develops. Ideally it is seen as a working document that the child and family can add to as needed. For example, after regulating through some angry feelings in therapy, the therapist might note that the child seemed to find the sandtray in the room calming and might suggest that the family use a small tray of sensory sand as a calming option at home. This strategy might be added as a suggestion to the child's plan, and the child and family can be encouraged to reflect on this the next time they come in for a session.

An example of a plan is provided below for your reference. As discussed, it is useful to develop these plans individually, adapting the language to suit the particular child and family. Talking with the family about where they can keep the plan and the form the plan should take is helpful. For example, older children might like to keep it as a note on their tablet or laptop, while for younger children a large sheet of paper, colorfully decorated and hung in a well-used area of the house might be the best option.

An example regulation plan

AMY'S PLAN

When my angry and upset feelings are beginning to get really big:

- My muscles get tense.

- It's hard to think properly.

- I want to be alone.

I can:

- Listen to music—my playlist.

- Read a book.

- Call my friends.

- Have some time in my room.

- Walk to Grandpa's, letting Mom know that's where I'm going.

- Call the helpline [include number].

My family can:

- Give me some space until I calm down.

- Leave me alone and not talk to me.

- Leave me to listen to my music for a bit.

If I'm really angry and upset I can:

- Call the helpline [include number].

- Go to the hospital [include name].

Other things I can try that might be calming:

- Having a shower.

- Doing some yoga stretches.

Legal and ethical responsibilities

As discussed, it is helpful to support grownups in a manner in which we would like them to support their child. While this means providing lots of nurturing and support, it also means that, at times, we need to be what Paris Goodyear-Brown (2021) refers to as a *safe boss*. We need to work in a way that keeps everyone safe, and this sometimes means involving child services so that the family is able to access further support.

It is essential that, as therapists, we are aware of our legal and ethical responsibilities in managing the risks associated with anger and emotional dysregulation. Given that reporting requirements vary between states and countries, and are different for therapists with different disciplines, the nature of these requirements will not be discussed here. What follows, however, is a discussion of how you can best navigate this space with children and families. Ensuring the family is aware of the limitations to confidentiality, maintaining a stance that they are doing their best, and being transparent around the process whenever possible can help support them through this.

Confidentiality is an important part of creating a safe space for children and families, and most therapists begin with an introduction around this early in therapy.

Acknowledging the limits to this in a developmentally appropriate way is essential; for a young child, this might be as simple as explaining that your job is to keep them safe and that if you can't do that you might need to tell someone about what is happening. Finding a balance here between acknowledging limitations and creating a space that feels welcoming is important, so keeping it simple and saying something like "If that happens, I will try to talk to you and your family about how we can manage that so that we can work through it together" is often helpful.

Families who are dealing with emotional regulation challenges are generally doing their best under really difficult circumstances. Acknowledging this often helps a family to feel held and supports them to share openly about what is happening, allowing you to better meet them where they are at. Importantly, you can acknowledge that a family is doing their best without condoning their behavior. For example, you might say something like "It sounds like it gets so hard when Amy does that. You find yourself getting angry too, despite your best efforts, and it can get unsafe."

Should a situation arise that requires you to notify child services, it is possible to explain to the family why it is necessary and share with them how you will do this. Knowing why you need to notify and what you will be saying is often reassuring for families and allows you to maintain the therapeutic relationship. Sometimes families may even wish to be present when you make the phone call and can feel reassured by you expressing some of the positive aspects, such as their willingness to engage in therapy and your commitment to working with them. This approach is often far preferable to notifying services without the family's knowledge, but this is not always possible. If the child is likely to be placed at further risk as a result of the family being aware of a notification, then it is essential that you do this without the family's knowledge.

A word about working online

Throughout this book I have offered suggestions around how therapeutic activities can be used online, recognizing that many therapists continue to work online having begun doing so during the Covid-19 pandemic and that many families find this to be an accessible option. There are, however, some important considerations in this space.

First, it is helpful to consider which children and families engage well online and which are best seen in the clinic. When families were unable to come into clinics, online sessions presented a next best option, which was crucial during the pandemic; however, as we move forward it is essential that we consider which families this works well for and which are better seen face to face. In addition to considering the preferences of families, sharing our clinical observations and recommendations is important.

Second, there are aspects around working with dysregulated children online that are necessary to consider. As discussed throughout this book, emotions can and do arise in the context of therapy sessions, and children who are quick to anger and become aggressive are likely to do so at some point in therapy. This often presents an opportunity to co-regulate the child and to support the grownup to do so, which can indeed be very helpful. It is essential to acknowledge, however, that your capacity for supporting regulation online is more limited. When working online you can only see the child's and grownup's faces and perhaps their shoulders and the upper part of their chest. This increases the likelihood that you may miss cues that indicate they are becoming dysregulated.

On a related point, when working online, therapists have far less control over the environment. Within the clinic setting you can ensure that the physical space is safe and can access the support of colleagues if a child or grownup begins engaging in aggressive or unsafe behavior. Online, you lack a knowledge of the child's surroundings and have no control of the physical environment. For example, if a child becomes angry and runs away from the screen you will lack any vision of what is happening and can do little to ensure their safety.

When you do work online, therefore, my recommendation would be that you do so only with children and families you have previously had the opportunity to meet face to face. Having a good sense of their triggers, knowing the signs that indicate they are becoming dysregulated and knowing what helps them to calm and how grownups are able to regulate them will support you to navigate online sessions more effectively. Talking with grownups around where sessions can be held within the house, ensuring that they will be present or close by should the child need support and establishing a plan around what you will all do if a child does escalate or if you have safety concerns during a session are all important. Having clear expectations around this ahead of time is essential.

A final consideration is that legal and ethical requirements vary within and across countries. If you are working with families in another state, it is essential that you are aware of your responsibilities and can follow the appropriate procedures if you do have concerns around safety.

CHAPTER 10

DEALING WITH COMMON TRIGGERS

HENRY

Henry was late to join an online session from school and was very angry that his teacher hadn't reminded him of it. When he connected with me, he demanded to know how he could get the 21 minutes he had missed back. I empathized with his feelings, remembering that things not going to plan was often very challenging for him. I gently explained that I couldn't extend the session and took some deep breaths along with Henry, acknowledging how hard this was for him. We spent some time with these feelings before I explained that I was worried that if we kept talking about this we wouldn't have time to do anything together. At this point Henry suggested a game of Connect 4 and we began to play. The game was regulating, and as the session progressed Henry and I were able to talk about those times when plans have to change, noticing this in the game and regulating as we did so. We were briefly able to relate this to Henry's day-to-day life.

Throughout this book I have tried to step you through a way of supporting children to regulate themselves, from helping them to understand and express anger, to supporting them to be curious about their anger, to developing calming strategies, to promoting an understanding of the role of thoughts in anger. The sequence is not necessarily linear and, in practice, there is often a circling back to earlier components, following the needs of the child and family. The sections up till now have been relevant for children who struggle with big feelings of anger, regardless of what might trigger those feelings. Therapists who are skilled in understanding children and families and adapting therapy accordingly will individualize the approaches and activities outlined. This work is often effective, and many children do not need to focus on their specific triggers.

Other children, however, will continue to struggle with those things that brought them to therapy in the first place. This might include perfectionism, managing when plans change or not having control over situations. Having developed a good understanding of anger and having built up their repertoire of coping skills, children are often in a better position to engage in this work. As in the example above, triggers can be addressed in a playful way. This chapter provides some activities that can be useful here as well as some thoughts about how grownups can support children in this space.

Once a child understands their anger and has developed some coping skills, therapy can be a useful space to practice using what they have learnt in the face of their triggers. In therapy we provide the scaffold, giving the child an opportunity to face what they find challenging with support, drawing on the strategies they have developed. The experience of practicing this in sessions helps children begin to develop a different way of responding, creating a new path. In the example above, the child who struggles when things don't go how he imagined is able to experience this in a titrated manner, with the support he needs to begin navigating it differently. As in all of the activities included in this chapter, play in this context provides an engaging and supported environment in which children are gently exposed to, and supported to manage, those things they find hard.

The activities in this chapter will help you explore some of the situations and experiences that might contribute to a child's anger, and a selection of activities address common triggers. When working on something that is a trigger for a child, whether that be around changing plans or embracing mistakes, one activity is unlikely to be sufficient, so you will need to use this in combination with other work. For example, the *Slimy messy mistakes* activity may be useful for a child along with some picture books on making mistakes and some of the activities from *Creative Ways to Help Children Manage Anxiety* (Zandt and Barrett 2021). Rather than providing a comprehensive approach, therefore, I have included these activities in this chapter in the hope that they provide you with an understanding of how triggers might be specifically addressed through play.

Grownups also have a key role in supporting children who struggle with these triggers. Throughout the book we have seen a focus on helping grownups attune to their child and understand their triggers. Activities such as *How stretched are you today?* (Chapter 5) and *What's bugging you?* (Chapter 2) aim to increase the child's and family's awareness of what the child finds difficult. Many grownups become quite skilled at scaffolding their child, making accommodations and environmental adjustments. This support is essential, particularly for children with developmental differences. As children get older and find themselves in more environments where they are less closely supported by grownups, they may also benefit from working specifically on those things they find challenging. For this reason, pairing environmental support with some work around those things a child finds challenging is often very helpful. Engaging grownups in these activities and helping them relate this to how they can support a child in their day-to-day life works well.

As therapists, we can also become quite skilled at supporting a child through those things they find triggering. Providing scaffolding and support is essential in therapy, so, for example, warning a child who struggles with change around upcoming transitions creates safety and allows us to address other therapeutic goals. If, however, the child is struggling with transitions in their day-to-day life and the family are seeking support with this, we also need to build a child's coping skills and then reduce the amount of support we provide around this in sessions, helping the child to regulate through this when they need to move from one activity to another. This gives the child the experience of managing these challenges in a different way and allows you to show grownups how their child might be supported to do so. When working with a child around triggers, therefore, do consider those that are likely to come up naturally in your session: allowing the time to work through these as they arise can be incredibly powerful. What follows are some activities that provide a playful way of addressing triggers.

Changing plans with Connect 4

This activity uses the board game Connect 4 to help children who find changes of plan difficult.

What you need
Connect 4 game.

Introducing this activity
Connect 4 is a simple game in which the objective is to get four pieces in a row before your opponent does so. Most children are happy to play this game, and as we do so I notice what is happening for me, relating this to my plan. For example, I might place a piece while sharing that I have a plan. Having communicated that I have a plan to the child, I can then notice when my plan needs to change. For example, I might say something like "Oh no, you've put your piece there and that has ruined my plan. That's frustrating."

Modeling some regulation at this time, such as taking a breath or engaging in some movement, as well as some coping thoughts, like "Hmm, time to think of a new plan" or "I'm sure I can think of another way" is often a helpful way of indirectly teaching the child some coping strategies in this space. Ensuring that what you model is a good fit for the child is important. For example, younger children will benefit from having you model simpler regulation strategies and coping thoughts. Having a simple coping thought that you repeat out loud and that can be used in a range of situations is often a good fit for this age group.

Some children may struggle with changing plans in the context of the game and are likely to benefit from having you support them to regulate in this context. Others may be able to manage this in the game, despite struggling in their day-to-day life, and can be supported to link the two. For example, you might notice that you could see them pause and consider a new plan, wondering if this is something they do at home or at school.

Considerations and adaptations
There are some online versions of this game that can be useful if you are working with children in this way.

Grownups can be encouraged to play the game too and notice the feelings that come up for them when they are required to change their plans. You might like to help them relate this to their child's experiences and consider how they can support their child in the moment. Encouraging them to use some of the language that has arisen in the session will also help to provide continuity and support the child to use the strategies in their day-to-day life.

Slimy messy mistakes

This activity is useful for children who are easily angered by mistakes. It gives the chance to explore what it means to make mistakes and explore why mistakes can be helpful.

What you need
Ingredients for your favorite slime recipe.

Introducing this activity
Slime is undeniably messy, and making it is even more so. Whichever of the many readily available recipes you choose, it involves mixing glue and other ingredients with a slime activator, such as liquid starch or borax. Rather than using a recipe, however, I use the ingredients for making slime, without having any specification around the quantities. I explain that I don't have a recipe and that we'll have to work it out.

Children might express frustration or anxiety around this, and some might suggest that you look up a recipe when you do this, which can be a good opportunity to notice and name feelings and model some regulation. This process is important as you continue through this activity. Throughout the process you might notice the temptation to rescue the child and give them direction about how to make the slime.

When the slime is not right, I will often label this as a mistake and reflect on what we have learnt from it. Doing this gently and in a collaborative manner, through saying something like "Hmm, you're right, it's not looking stretchy enough. So, what does that tell us?" is often helpful. The child might, for example, learn that too much shaving cream makes the slime too solid, while too much glue makes it too sticky.

It can be really helpful to notice grownups' responses in this space too. Some may be very uncomfortable about the mistakes and you might notice the urge they have to jump in and fix it for the child. Helping grownups explore their own feelings and thoughts about this is often helpful.

Considerations and adaptations
Adjusting the slime until it looks and feels just right is a wonderfully messy experience. When reflecting on this with the child and their grownups, it is helpful to get curious about the feelings and thoughts that came up for them as they were making the slime. You can wonder about the way in which mistakes helped them learn about making slime. Talking more generally about how mistakes help us learn and encouraging the family to celebrate the learning that comes from mistakes in their day-to-day life is helpful.

Holding on to the shoulds

Sometimes children have very strong thoughts in the form of *shoulds* that they hold on to tightly. Situations that challenge these thoughts can make them anxious and angry. This activity is useful for those children and helps them to explore the idea of holding thoughts more loosely. Because this activity focuses on thoughts, it is one that I use with older children. The activity was inspired by Dion's (2018) discussion of how our unrealistic expectations or "shoulds" can cause us to become dysregulated and by the Pushing Away Paper exercise in Russ Harris's ACT Made Simple (2019).

What you need

Small pieces of cardboard and some markers or some symbols, toys and figures that the child can choose from.

Introducing this activity

I begin this activity by noticing a should thought the child has, such as "I should do really well at school" or "Everyone should like me." I comment that I can see that this thought is one they are holding on really tight to and ask if we can explore this. I invite them either to find something in the clinic room that might symbolize this thought for them or to write it on a piece of card. For example, a child might choose a sandtray miniature of a teacher to indicate that they should always do well at school. If the child has chosen something to symbolize the thought I will express a curiosity about what they chose, which might lead to some helpful discussion.

Once we have something to hold, I encourage them to hold it as tightly as they possibly can with both hands and we agree on a time frame that they will try to do so for. For example, children might have me count to 30 while they hold the should thought really tightly or we might agree to set a timer for a minute or so. I may also share one of my should thoughts and hold it in a similar way. It can also be helpful to encourage the child's grownups to share a should thought of their own and hold it in the same manner.

When holding the should thought I often exaggerate my response, using my face and body to express the strain of holding this so tightly. I notice what happens with the child and grownup as they hold their should thoughts too, and we share some reflections on what it was like to do so after the allotted time. Exploring what the child noticed about the way their body responded, how they felt when holding the should thought tightly and the sorts of thoughts they found themselves having can all be helpful.

We then practice holding the should thought loosely, perhaps resting it lightly on one hand. We repeat this for the allotted time and again notice how this feels, comparing the two. It can also be fun to extend this experience. For example, you might explore a child's capacity for thought by having them solve math problems while holding tightly and then more loosely or check out their capacity to do something like hop on one leg while holding tightly and then more loosely.

When reflecting on this activity, it is helpful to explain that we can hold our should thoughts more or less tightly. Holding them tightly means being very focused on these thoughts and often makes it hard for us to focus on or do other things. Holding these should thoughts more loosely often frees us up to be able to think more clearly and to do other things. You can also get curious about whether the should thought is something that they want to hold on to or whether it might be something they might want to put down. Some children will want to replace the should thought with something more realistic, such as "I try my best at school" or "Not everyone has to like me."

Considerations and adaptations

Reflecting on what these should thoughts mean in the child's day-to-day life and how they might be able to hold these thoughts more lightly is often helpful. Grownups can also be supported to help children reflect on this in the moment, using prompts such as "Wow! You are really holding that should thought super tight right now. That can be tiring. Could we loosen our grip on it a bit?"

Some children might decide that they do want to loosen their grip and would prefer to keep the item somewhere else, such as on a shelf somewhere at home. Encouraging them to do so is often helpful and can be a good reminder of the discussion.

While this activity is useful for older children and grownups it is not appropriate for younger children, many of whom will struggle to articulate their thoughts and find the concepts in this activity too complex.

Final Thoughts

Writing the *Creative Ways* series has been a journey, one I feel privileged to have shared with the wonderful Suzanne Barrett and with our amazing workshop participants and readers. My own development as a therapist also continues to be a journey, one which I see reflected in these pages. The work we undertake is so important that embracing our own ongoing learning can feel extremely uncomfortable, and I often wish I knew 20 years ago what I know now. Inevitably though, our development continues over time with ongoing learning and reflection deepening our skills. Welcoming this growth facilitates our development, both as therapists and as human beings.

As you reach the end of this book, I would encourage you to pause and reflect. Notice what you are drawn to, as well as what you feel challenged by. Lean in to those feelings and get curious about how this might relate to your practice, your training and experience to date, and your own therapeutic style. Reflect too on how these responses relate to your own experience of anger and regulation. Consider what you might incorporate into your practice and notice those areas where you might want to grow or develop, pondering how you might do so. Identifying some initial steps you can take often helps to begin the journey toward bigger changes. Be kind to yourself, remembering that it takes time to walk a new path, and seek out those who can guide you along the way.

Thank you for all of the work you do with children and their families. This work is incredibly challenging at times and requires us to give so much of ourselves. It is also very powerful, with impacts that ripple well beyond what we can observe in the moment. Trust in the ripples.

Keep playing and learning,

Fiona

Creative Child Therapy Workshops
https://childpsychologyworkshops.com.au

References

Alderson-Day, B. and Fernyhough, C. (2015) 'Inner speech: Development, phenomenology, and neurobiology.' *Psychological Bulletin 141*, 5, 931–965.

American Psychiatric Association (2013) *Diagnostic and Statistical Manual of Mental Disorders* (5th edn). Washington, DC: American Psychiatric Association.

Bell, M.A. (2020) 'Mother–child behavioral and physiological synchrony.' *Advances in Child Development and Behavior 58*, 163–188.

Berkout, O.V., Tinsley, D. and Flynn, M.K. (2020) 'A review of anger, hostility, and aggression from an ACT Perspective.' *Journal of Contextual Behavioral Science 11*, 34–43.

Bertie, L., Johnston, K. and Lill, S. (2021) 'Parent emotion socialisation of young children and the mediating role of emotion regulation.' *Australian Journal of Psychology 73*, 3, 293–305.

Black, T. (2022) *ACT for Treating Children: The Essential Guide to Acceptance and Commitment Therapy for Kids.* Oakland, CA: New Harbinger.

Braet, C., Theuwis, L., Van Durme, K., Vandewalle, J. *et al.* (2014) 'Emotion regulation in children with emotional problems.' *Cognitive Therapy and Research 38*, 5, 493–504.

Carlson, G.A., Singh, M.K., Amaya-Jackson, L., Benton, T.D. *et al.* (2023) 'Narrative review: Impairing emotional outbursts: What they are and what we should do about them.' *Journal of the American Academy of Child and Adolescent Psychiatry 62*, 2, 135–150.

Carreras, J., Carter, A.S., Heberle, A., Forbes, D. and Gray, S.O. (2019) 'Emotion regulation and parent distress: Getting at the heart of sensitive parenting among parents of preschool children experiencing high sociodemographic risk.' *Journal of Child and Family Studies 28*, 11, 2953–2962.

Child Development Institute (2016) *Navigating the Middle Years with Self-control: Stop Now and Pause.* Available at https://childdevelop.ca/snap/sites/default/files/CDI%20SNAP%20Booklet%202016%20FINAL.pdf

Clifford, P., Gevers, C., Jonkman, K.M., Boer, F. and Begeer S. (2022) 'The effectiveness of an attention-based intervention for school-aged autistic children with anger regulating problems: A randomized controlled trial.' *Autism Research 15*, 10, 1971–1984.

Coghill, D., Banaschewski, T., Cortese, S., Asherson, P. *et al.* (2021) 'The management of ADHD in children and adolescents: Bringing evidence to the clinic: Perspective from the European ADHD Guidelines Group (EAGG).' *European Child and Adolescent Psychiatry.* https://doi.org/10.1007/s00787-021-01871-x

Day, C. and Day, R. (2012) *Matryoshkas in Therapy: Creative Ways to Use Russian Dolls with Clients.* Rugby: Brook Creative Therapy.

Delahooke, M. (2020) *Beyond Behaviour: Using Brain Science and Compassion to Understand and Solve Children's Behavioural Challenges.* London: John Murray Press.

Dion, L. (2018) *Aggression in Play Therapy: A Neurobiological Approach for Integrating Intensity.* New York, NY: W.W. Norton.

Fuggle, P., Dunsmuir, S. and Curry, V. (2013) *CBT with Children, Young People and Families.* London: Sage.

Garland, A.F., Hawley, K.M., Brookman-Frazee, L. and Hurlburt, M.S. (2008) 'Identifying common elements for evidence-based psychosocial treatments for children's disruptive behavior problems.' *Journal of the American Academy of Child and Adolescent Psychiatry 47*, 5, 505–514.

Girard, L.C. (2021) 'Concomitant trajectories of internalising, externalising, and peer problems across childhood: A person-centered approach.' *Research on Child and Adolescent Psychopathology 49*, 12, 1551–1565.

Goodyear-Brown, P. (2010) *Play Therapy with Traumatized Children: A Prescriptive Approach.* Hoboken, NJ: John Wiley and Sons.

Goodyear-Brown, P. (2021) *Parents as Partners in Child Therapy: A Clinician's Guide.* New York, NY: The Guilford Press.

Gottman, J. and Declaire, J. (1997) *Raising an Emotionally Intelligent Child: The Heart of Parenting.* New York, NY: Simon and Schuster.

Gottman, J., Katz, L.F. and Hooven, C. (1996) 'Parental meta-emotion philosophy and the emotional life of families: Theoretical models and preliminary data.' *Journal of Family Psychology 10*, 3, 243–268.

Greenberg, L.S. (2002) *Emotion-Focused Therapy: Coaching Clients to Work Through Their Feelings.* Washington, DC: American Psychological Association.

Greene, R. (2014) *Lost at School: Why Our Kids at School with Behavioral Challenges Are Falling Through the Cracks and How We Can Help Them.* New York, NY: Scribner.

Gruhn, M.A. and Compas, B.E. (2020) 'Effects of maltreatment on coping and emotion regulation in childhood and adolescence: A meta-analytic review.' *Child Abuse & Neglect 103*, 104446 https://doi.org/10.1016/j.chiabu.2020.104446

Hajal, N.J. and Paley, B. (2020) 'Parental emotion and emotion regulation: A critical target of study for research and intervention to promote child emotion socialization.' *Developmental Psychology 56*, 3, 403–417.

Harmon, S.L., Stephens, H.F., Repper, K.K., Driscoll, K.A. and Kistner, J.A. (2019) 'Children's rumination to sadness and anger: Implications for depression and aggression.' *Journal of Clinical Child and Adolescent Psychology 48*, 622–632.

Harris, R. (2019) *ACT Made Simple: An Easy-to-Read Primer on Acceptance and Commitment Therapy* (2nd edn). Oakland, CA: New Harbinger.

Havighurst, S. and Kehoe, C. (2017) 'The Role of Parental Emotion Regulation in Parental Emotion Socialization: Implications for Intervention.' In K. Deater-Deckard and R. Panneton (eds.) *Parental Stress and Early Child Development: Adaptive and Maladaptive Outcomes* (pp.285–307). Cham: Springer International.

Hoffman, K., Cooper, G., Powell, B. and Benton, C.M. (2017) *Raising a Secure Child: How Circle of Security Parenting Can Help You Nurture Your Child's Attachment, Emotional Resilience and Freedom to Explore.* New York, NY: The Guilford Press.

Holmberg Bergman, T., Renhorn, E., Berg, B., Lappalainen, P., Ghaderi, A. and Hirvikoski, T. (2023) 'Acceptance and commitment therapy group intervention for parents of children with disabilities (Navigator ACT): An open feasibility trial.' *Journal of Autism and Developmental Disorders 53*, 5, 1834–1849.

Hughes, D., Golding, K. and Hudson, J. (2019) *Healing Relational Trauma with Attachment-Focused Interventions: Dyadic Developmental Psychotherapy with Children and Families.* New York, NY: W.W. Norton.

Kazdin, A.E. (2017) 'Parent Management Training and Problem-Solving Skills Training for Child and Adolescent Conduct Problems.' In J.R. Weisz and A.E. Kazdin (eds.) *Evidence-Based Psychotherapies for Children and Adolescents* (pp.142–158). New York, NY: The Guilford Press.

Lachman, J.E., Boxmeyer, C.L., Gilpin, A.T. and Powell, N.P. (2021) 'Cognitive-Behavioral Intervention for Aggressive Children: The Anger Coping and Coping Power Programs.' In M.E. Feinberg (ed.) *Designing Evidence-Based Public Health and Prevention Programs: Expert Program Developers Explain the Science and Art* (pp.9–21). New York, NY: Routledge.

Landreth, G. (2023) *Play Therapy: The Art of the Relationship* (4th edn). New York, NY: Routledge.

Lavi, I., Katz, L.F., Ozer, E.J. and Gross, J.J. (2019) 'Emotion reactivity and regulation in maltreated children: A meta-analysis.' *Child Development 90*, 5, 1503–1524.

Li, S., Ma, X. and Zhang, Y. (2023) 'Intergenerational transmission of aggression: A meta-analysis of relationship between interparental conflict and aggressive behavior of children and youth.' *Current Psychology* [Advance online publication]. https://doi.org/10.1007/s12144-022-04219-z

Matthys, W. and Schutter, D.J.L.G. (2021) 'Increasing effectiveness of cognitive behavioral therapy for conduct problems in children and adolescents: What can we learn from neuroimaging studies?' *Clinical Child and Family Psychology Review 24*, 484–499.

McQuillan, M.E. and Bates, J.E. (2017) 'Parental Stress and Child Temperament.' In K. Deater-Deckard and R. Panneton (eds.) *Parental Stress and Early Child Development: Adaptive and Maladaptive Outcomes* (pp.75–106). Cham: Springer International Publishing.

Miller, W.R. and Moyers, T.B. (2021) *Effective Psychotherapists: Clinical Skills That Improve Client Outcome.* New York, NY: The Guilford Press.

Morales, S., Tang, A., Bowers, M.E., Miller, N.V. *et al.* (2022) 'Infant temperament prospectively predicts general psychopathology in childhood.' *Developmental Psychopathology 34*, 3, 774–783.

Morris A.S., Silk J.S., Steinberg L., Myers S.S. and Robinson L.R. (2007) 'The role of the family context in the development of emotion regulation.' *Social Development 16*, 2, 361–388.

Perepletchikova, F., Nathanson, D., Axelrod, S.R., Merrill, C. *et al.* (2017) 'Randomized clinical trial of dialectical behavior therapy for preadolescent children with disruptive mood dysregulation disorder: Feasibility and outcomes.' *Journal of the American Academy of Child and Adolescent Psychiatry 56*, 10, 832–840.

Porges, S. (2017) *The Pocket Guide to the Polyvagal Theory: The Transformative Power of Feeling Safe.* New York, NY: W.W. Norton.

Powell, N.P., Lochman, J.E., Boxmeyer, C.L., Barry, T.D. and Pardini, D.A. (2017) 'The Coping Power Program for Aggressive Behavior in Children.' In J.R. Weisz and A.E. Kazdin (eds.) *Evidence-Based Psychotherapies for Children and Adolescents* (pp.159–176). New York, NY: The Guilford Press.

Rathus, J.H. and Miller, A.L. (2015) *DBT Skills Manual for Adolescents.* New York, NY: The Guilford Press.

Rowling, J.K. (2007) *Harry Potter and the Deathly Hallows.* London: Bloomsbury.

Rubenstein, L. (2013) *Visiting Feelings.* Washington, DC: Magination Press.

Schaefer, C.E. and Drewes, A.A. (2014) *The Therapeutic Powers of Play: 20 Core Agents of Change* (2nd edn). Hoboken, NJ: John Wiley & Sons.

Siegel, D. (2012) *The Whole-Brain Child: 12 Revolutionary Strategies to Nurture Your Child's Developing Mind.* London: Robinson.

Siegel, D. (2020) *The Developing Mind: How Relationships and the Brain Interact and Shape Who We Are* (3rd edn). New York, NY: The Guilford Press.

Škėrienė S. & Jucevičienė P. (2020) 'Problem solving through values: A challenge for thinking and capability development.' *Thinking Skills and Creativity 37*, 100694. https://doi.org/10.1016/j.tsc.2020.100694

Smith, J. (2022) *Why Has No One Ever Told Me This Before?* London: Penguin.

Smith, J., Kyle, R.G., Daniel, B. and Hubbard, G. (2018) 'Patterns of referral and waiting times for specialist Child and Adolescent Mental Health Services.' *Child and Adolescent Mental Health 23*, 1, 43–49.

Smith, S.D., Stephens, H.F., Repper, K. and Kistner, J.A. (2016) 'The relationship between anger rumination and aggression in typically developing children and high-risk adolescents.' *Journal of Psychopathology and Behavioral Assessment 38*, 515–527.

Somerville, M.P., MacIntyre, H., Harrison, A. and Mauss, I.G. (2023) 'Emotion controllability beliefs and young people's anxiety and depression symptoms: A systematic review.' *Adolescent Research Review.* https://doi.org/10.1007/s40894-023-00213-z

Stefan, C.A. and Negrean, D. (2021) 'Parent- and teacher-rated emotion regulation strategies in relation to preschoolers' attachment representations: A longitudinal perspective.' *Review of Social Development 31*, 3, 180–195.

Tan, P.Z., Oppenheimer, C.W., Ladouceur, C.D., Butterfield, R.D. and Silk, J.S. (2020) 'A review of associations between parental emotion socialization behaviors and the neural substrates of emotional reactivity and regulation in youth.' *Developmental Psychology 56*, 3, 516–527.

Thöne, AK., Dose, C., Junghänel, M., Hautmann, C. *et al.* (2023) 'Identifying symptoms of ADHD and disruptive behavior disorders most strongly associated with functional impairment in children: A symptom-level approach.' *Journal of Psychopathology and Behavioral Assessment 45*, 277–293.

Treisman, K. (2017) *A Therapeutic Treasure Box for Working with Children and Adolescents with Developmental Trauma: Creative Techniques and Activities.* London: Jessica Kingsley Publishers.

Treisman, K. (2020) *Binnie the Baboon: Anxiety and Stress Activity Book.* London: Jessica Kingsley Publishers.

Van den Akker, A.L., Hoffenaar, P. and Overbeek, G. (2022) 'Temper tantrums in toddlers and preschoolers: Longitudinal associations with adjustment problems.' *Journal of Developmental and Behavioral Pediatrics 43*, 7, 409–417.

Van Rest, M.M., Van Nieuwenhijzen, M., Kupersmidt, J.B., Vriens, A., Schuengel, C. and Mattys, W. (2020) 'Accidental and ambiguous situations reveal specific social information processing biases and deficits in adolescents with low intellectual level and clinical levels of externalizing behavior.' *Journal of Abnormal Child Psychology 48*, 1411–1424.

Vygotsky, L.S. (1986) *Thought and Language*. Translated by A. Kozulin. Cambridge, MA: Massachusetts Institute of Technology Press. (Original work published 1954)

Wesselhoeft, R., Stringaris, A., Sibbersen, C., Kristensen, R.V., Bojesen, A.B. and Talait, A. (2019) 'Dimensions and subtypes of oppositionality and their relation to comorbidity and psychosocial characteristics.' *European Child and Adolescent Psychiatry 28*, 3, 351–365.

Yasenik, L. and Gardner, K. (2012) *Play Therapy Dimensions Model: A Decision-Making Guide for Integrative Play Therapists*. London: Jessica Kingsley Publishers.

Zandt, F. and Barrett, S. (2017) *Creative Ways to Help Children Manage Big Feelings: A Therapist's Guide to Working with Preschool and Primary Children*. London: Jessica Kingsley Publishers.

Zandt, F. and Barrett, S. (2021) *Creative Ways to Help Children Manage Anxiety: Ideas and Activities for Working Therapeutically with Worried Children and Their Families*. London: Jessica Kingsley Publishers.